平衡

balance walking™

PRESIDENT'S CHALLENGE PROGRAM

*Balance Walking is a proud advocate of the President's Challenge Physical Activity and Fitness Program.*

**www.presidentschallenge.org**

Balance Walking



ISBN 978-0-615-19088-4

# Dedication

I would like to dedicate this book to my wife Angela who has accepted me and my workaholic pace and lifestyle. Thank you for understanding what drives me.

To my three daughters, Kerrin, Raina and Bella, all special in their own way and each one a joy to my life.

Mom and dad, you are very much missed. Thank you for being you.

# To My Readers

If you have picked this book up and thumbed through the pages, I request just one thing. Give yourself 15 minutes each day for 3 months. If you don't feel more alive, more energetic, younger, and if your friends and family have not noticed a difference in you; then please email me and I will have one of our coaches personally contact you to review what you are doing and how we can help you.

I am a dedicated workaholic and love what I do and just do not have enough time in the day to get everything done, EVERY DAY.

This started out as a program to help me change my lifestyle, to lose weight, increase my energy level and look better, etc. I know it works, I have seen its effects on hundreds of people.

If this book can help you change your lifestyle then I will have shared something special with you. Remember this is not a quick fix, it is about changing your lifestyle for the rest of your life for just 15 minutes a day. It is a small investment for a fuller, healthier, happier life.

Notice

This book is intended as a reference and introduction only, not as a medical manual. The information presented is not a medical manual and this information is not a substitute for any treatment that may have been prescribed by your doctor. If you think you have medical issues or problems you should always see a doctor.



Understand that you are solely responsible for the way this information is perceived and utilized and do so at your own risk. In no way will the author be responsible for injuries or other problems that might occur due to the use of this material or any actions taken based on the content of this material. The author will not be held responsible for the conduct of any companies and websites recommended within this book.

Mention of companies, organizations or authorities does not imply that they have endorsed this book or the author.

Now that we have gotten this out of the way let's get out there and live life to the fullest.

# Acknowlegments

I wish to acknowledge a number of people whose help and contributions made this book possible.

To all members of my family who have accepted me and my workaholic pace and lifestyle, thank you.

Every book is built on input and contributions developed over time for everyone who has helped and contributed to my journey through life and experience, thank you.

Special thanks to Coach Sue Bozgoz for her tireless support and input. Donna Robertson, Sports Pedorthist specialist, Dr. William Faddock DPM, C.Ped, Dr. Craig Aaron, Chiropractor, author and yoga specialist for developing simple yoga routines for Balance walking, my assistant Alison Strohfus for the many retypes, Melissa Schultheiss for artwork and editing contribution and Hania Whitfield for reviews and editing suggestions and to Dr. Karl Schwanbeck for his personal Nordic pole walking training and input on the many Nordic pole walking programs in Germany and Jeff Hopeck for designing a Kettlebell routine specifically for Balance walking. For anyone I have missed my apologies.

# Table of Contents

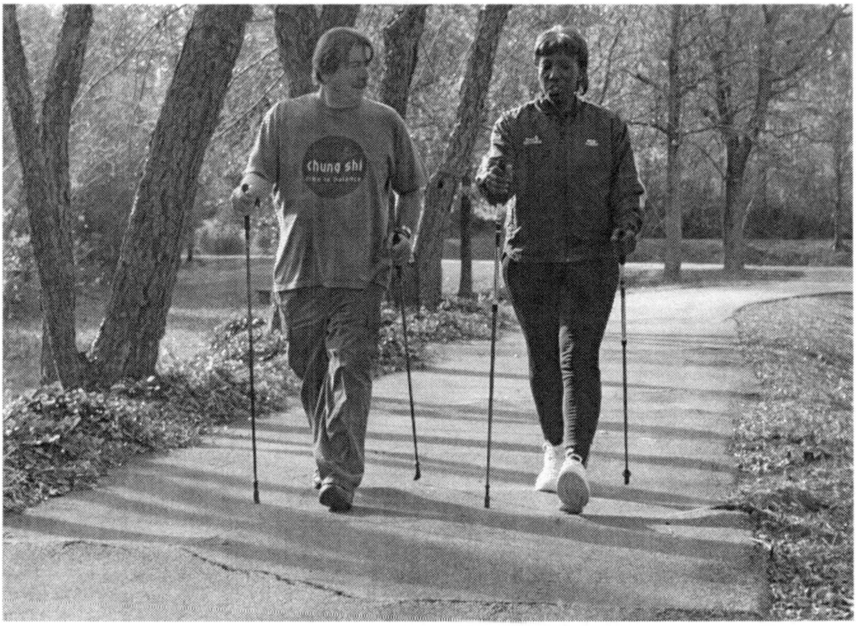


Author Ray Margiano and Millie Daniels, Nordic pole walking master coach and trainer

## Balance Walking – A Way of Life

### A Low-Impact Activity for Everyone

### Busy Lifestyles – A Great Solution

Daily exercise, one of the essential components for good health, is fun and easy with the Balance Walking way. Simply stated, Balance walking increases your benefits in reduced time. Time is the key factor that will impact whatever you pursue, which is why it is so critical to choose some form of activity you can do anywhere, anytime, and easily blending it into your lifestyle.

# Walking

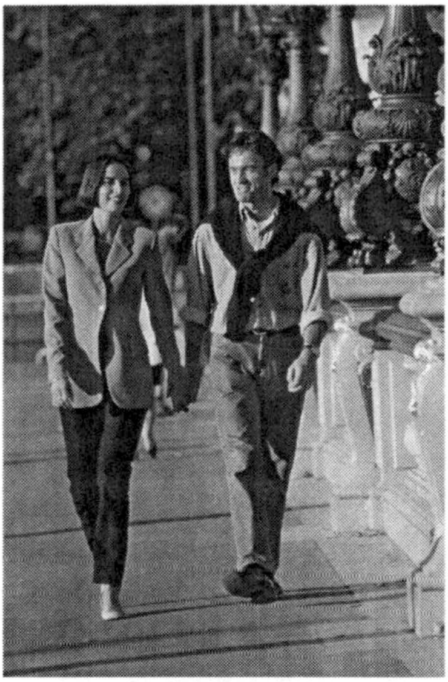

Did you know... The average person walks the equivalent distance of 3.5 times around the world during their lifetime!

Walking is the world's oldest and most popular form of exercise with the least amount of strain, on the body.

Unfortunately, most people do not receive the full potential benefits from their walks, and see little improvement over time. In addition, most people think it is boring and too time-consuming.

Walking has just been given a shot of adrenaline that has taken this simple exercise to a new level! Through the combination of today's technology and years of accumulated knowledge on walking techniques, we have created Balance Walking. Walking has become more fun with the simple addition of two components, walking poles and Chung Shi specialty shoes. With the Balance Walking System you get more of a workout for every fitness level, with less time. You'll work up to 90% of your muscles while you walk using the Balance Walking System. Although you are using more muscles, Balance Walking is natural. There is no strain on the body, but you are able to increase your calorie burn up to 50% compared to regular walking. This means that people with time constraints can get sufficient results in less time.

Pole walking gives you an upper-body workout while you walk. It builds arm, shoulder and back muscles while reducing tension in your shoulders, neck and back. It also gets your heart pumping, allowing you to reach your target heart-rate without the negative impact that running has on your body. This means more calorie burn and improved cardiovascular performance while using up to 90% of your muscles.

Chung Shi specialty shoes are uniquely designed to work your core muscles, toning and strengthening your abs, muscles, buttocks and back. They force better posture and target under-utilized muscles, building more muscle mass and in turn increasing calorie consumption. They may also improve or reduce varicose veins and the appearance of cellulite and ultimately help stomp out fat.

The components that make up this breakthrough in exercise have been thoroughly tested and validated, providing much documentation and studies to support the individual components of Balance Walking and its benefits.

Balance Walking has been created to bring basic fundamental, well-proven concepts together to introduce you to a lifestyle change you can enjoy and easily accomplish for the rest of your life.

Just devote a minimum of 15 minutes a day to Balance Walking and you and your friends will notice the difference.

## No More Excuses

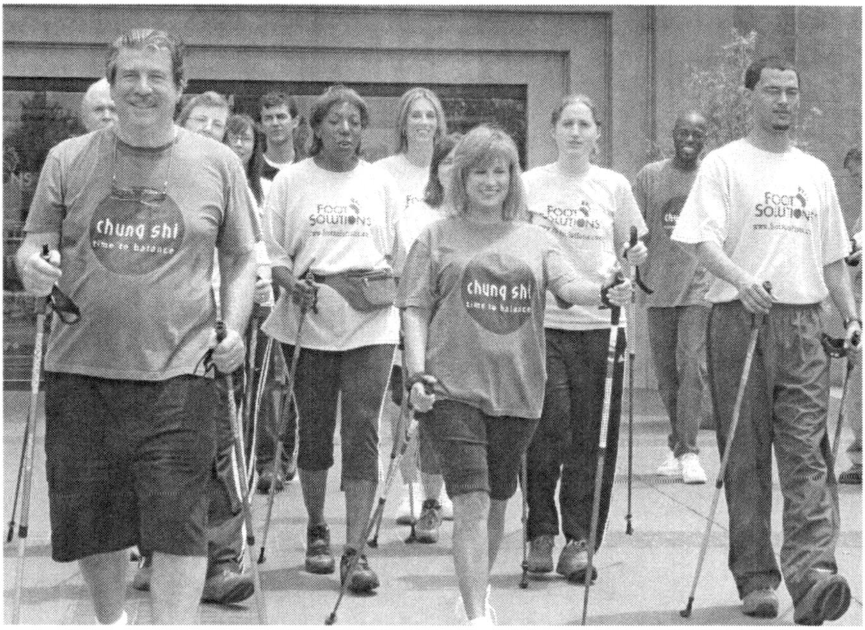


1. IT'S TOO HARD!

Balance Walking is low impact, less stressful than jogging, with 50% more calorie burn than regular walking.

2. I DON'T HAVE TIME!

With only 15 minutes per day the Balance Walking Program is designed to give you more benefits in less time using proven concepts.

3. EXERCISE IS ROUTINE AND BORING!

Balance Walking is a combination of simple, efficient, proven concepts that offers you an easy way to change your lifestyle. The primary concept is based on Nordic Pole Walking, simple stress reduction sessions, flexibility, maintenance, basic muscle toning/shaping and healthy eating habits. They can be done alone or as a social activity with a group or trainer.

4. CAN'T GET TO THE GYM!

Balance Walking can be done anywhere, anytime and is very inexpensive.

## GET BACK IN THE GAME

With Balance Walking it is all about you.

- For 15 minutes a day, it is just you.
- You can fulfill your own potential.
- How far and how long you go is up to you.
- How fast you go is up to you.
- No one is chasing you; it is your body and your mind. Get 50% more benefits over regular walking without feeling additional exertion.

If you want to drink from the fountain of youth, if you are interested in anti-aging benefits and a slew of things you will feel better about, then make this 15 minute commitment and live a fuller, more active life.

The Chinese have a saying that 10,000 steps per day lead to a healthy mind and healthy body. Through the use of Nordic Pole Walking and Foot Solutions' specially designed shoes used for the Balance Walking program, you can reduce this number down to 5,000 steps per day and get similar benefits. This is a 50% savings in time; the one element that impacts most people and most programs.

1. Dr. Cedric Bryant, Chief Science Officer for The American Council on Exercise (ACE) states "It's so low impact and joint friendly, and it's a relatively simple way of taking what many people are already doing, walking, and boosting it up a notch to burn extra calories." – The Wall Street Journal, 2/1/07.

2. "As a trainer and athlete, I am amazed with Balance Walking. Regardless of your age, you can walk to good health. You use 90% of your muscles, it is low-impact and you can have fun while exercising. I have clients with Parkinson's and other medical conditions who have difficulty walking. With the Nordic poles they are now walking with better posture and able to work out with more intensity. I have another client who has lost 12 pounds in 6 weeks of Balance Walking. I can't say enough!" – Karen J. Iverson RN, CPT, CFT, Fitness Practitioner, CHN, Balance Walking Master Instructor.

3. Cooper Institute Study Summary, September, 2002, validates calorie burn as well as no perceived increase in exertion.

The Cooper Institute in Texas compared physiological responses of Nordic Walking to regular walking. The calorie expenditure and the oxygen consumption increased an average of 20%, and the heart-rate increased with 10 beats per minute when using the Nordic Walking poles. The interesting thing is that even though the body works harder using the poles, the RPE (rated perceived exertion) was the same walking with or without poles.

Dr. Tim Church said, "Some individuals increased as much as 46% in oxygen consumption and just about the same in calorie expenditure."

Quotes from study:

"Individuals who poled more intensely had higher oxygen consumption."

"There is potential for considerably more or less benefit depending on the selection of poling-off intensity. This may have particular significance for individuals who need to increase calorie expenditure but have walking speed limitations."

"Increased calorie expenditure, with no corresponding increase in perceived exertion during Nordic Walking, may have important public health applications."

## The 4 Pillars of Balance Walking

Balance Walking combines the 4 pillars of health with complimentary elements that produce a synergistic effect unlike any other single program of its kind. It is the blend of activities and disciplines that will help restore and rejuvenate your life and energy; all in just 15 minutes a day.

Balance Walking is about changing the way you live simply and easily to help guide you into a more healthful and balanced lifestyle. Achieving physical fitness alone is not the solution. The formulation for a balanced lifestyle includes: fitness/aerobic plus strength/muscle mass plus flexibility/stress management reduction and healthy eating (no dieting). Balance Walking provides a full foundation from which to face the day to day stresses of life, not only for survival purposes but to help you lead a very active full life for the rest of your life.

### Balance Walking

The "Balance Walking Movement" is a Fit for Life program that involves a complete system to help you adjust to a lifestyle that is right for a healthier, more active you, with as little as fifteen minutes per day.

Benefits of Balance Walking

- Helps you look and feel years younger
- Burn up to 50% more calories than traditional walking
- Strengthens core muscles – tone abs, buttocks, and back muscles
- Reduces stress to knees, hips and back up to 30%
- Increases strength and endurance
- Enhances cardiovascular performance up to 22%
- Improves posture and body alignment.
- Relieves pain and tension in neck, shoulders and back
- Connects mind, body & spirit, promoting a positive healthy lifestyle
- Increases circulation in feet and legs
- Improves respiration
- Activates foot reflexology zones
- May improve or reduce varicose veins
- Reduces appearance of cellulite
- Improves balance and performance
- Reduces weight
- Reduces tension
- Improves overall health and fitness

**Make a 15 minute a day commitment!**

## Activity Goal

Commit to just 15 minutes per day of moderate intensity of physical activity based on your current level of fitness.

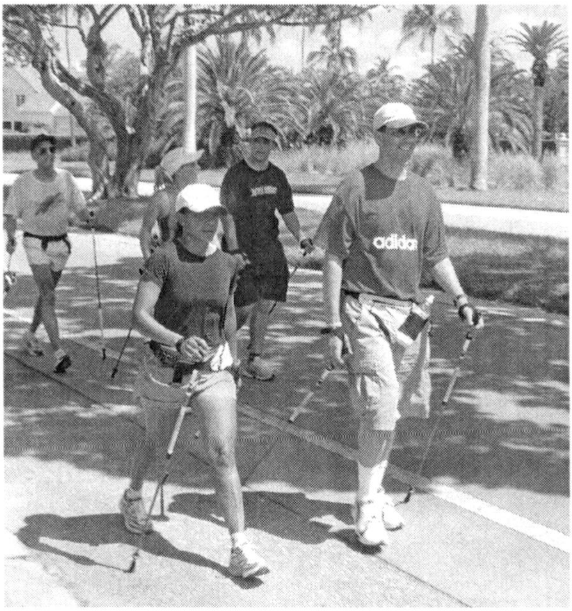

## The Secret of Staying Motivated

Part of our Balance Walking Plan is to help you stay motivated. The secret to staying motivated is to form a realistic physical fitness goal. For example, committing to 15 minutes per day, everyday is achievable and realistic. Each day after your activity, keep track by logging your minutes using the Presidents Challenge program, Balance Walking: (http://www.balancewalking.com). We have found that it is a great way to accumulate and chart progress and create excitement and camaraderie among Balance Walking groups. Balance Walking groups can also compete against each other or as teams; check the

Balance Walking website for a Balance Walking coach or group in your area and for free introductory classes located near you. Attending group walks and events will improve your form and help keep you motivated to accomplish your personal goals.

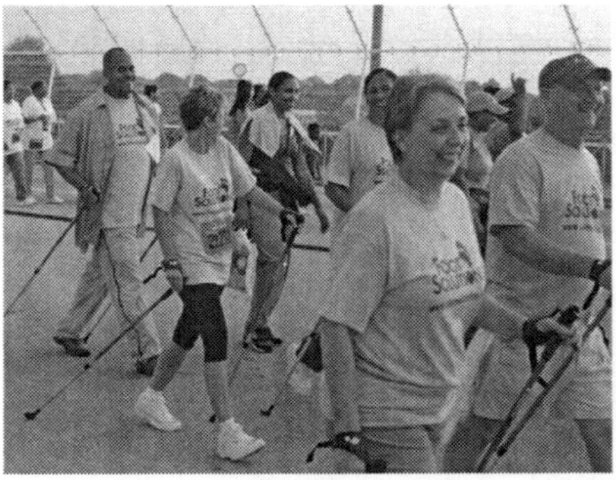
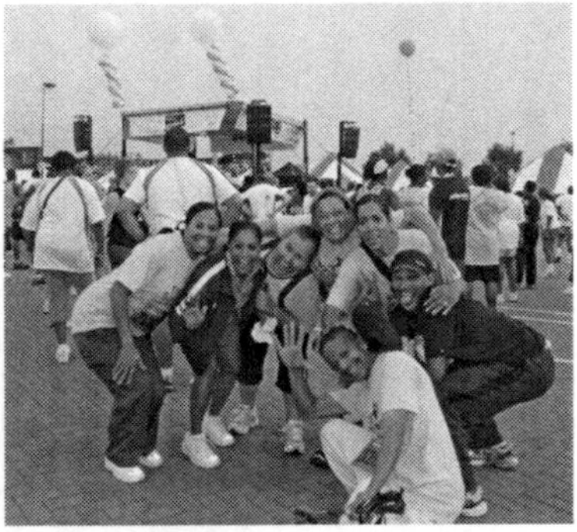

Social Events/Race Walks

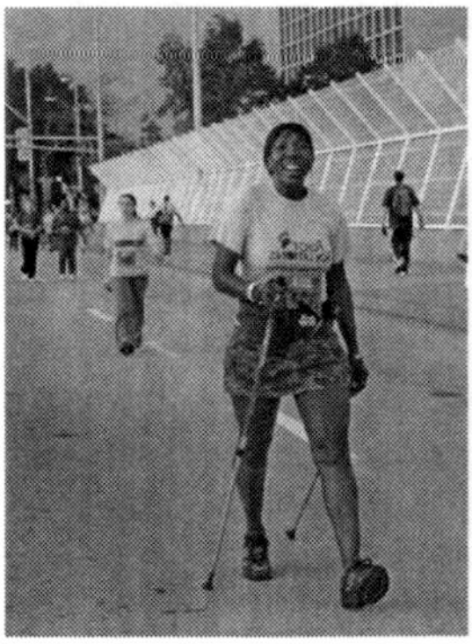
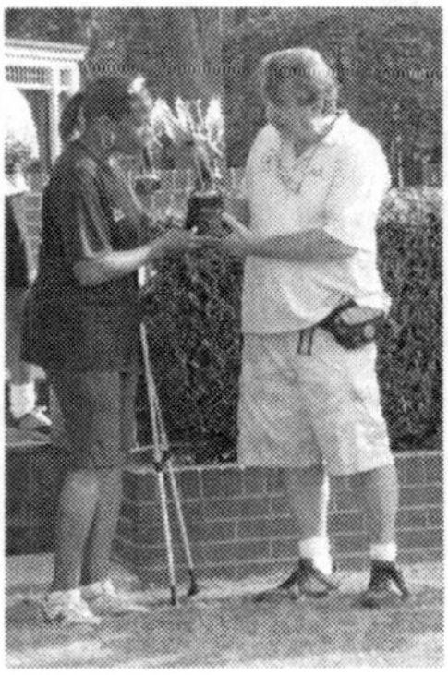
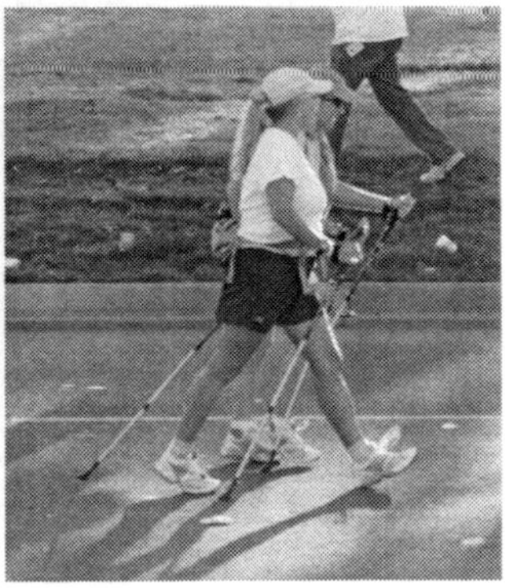

Organized Race Walking

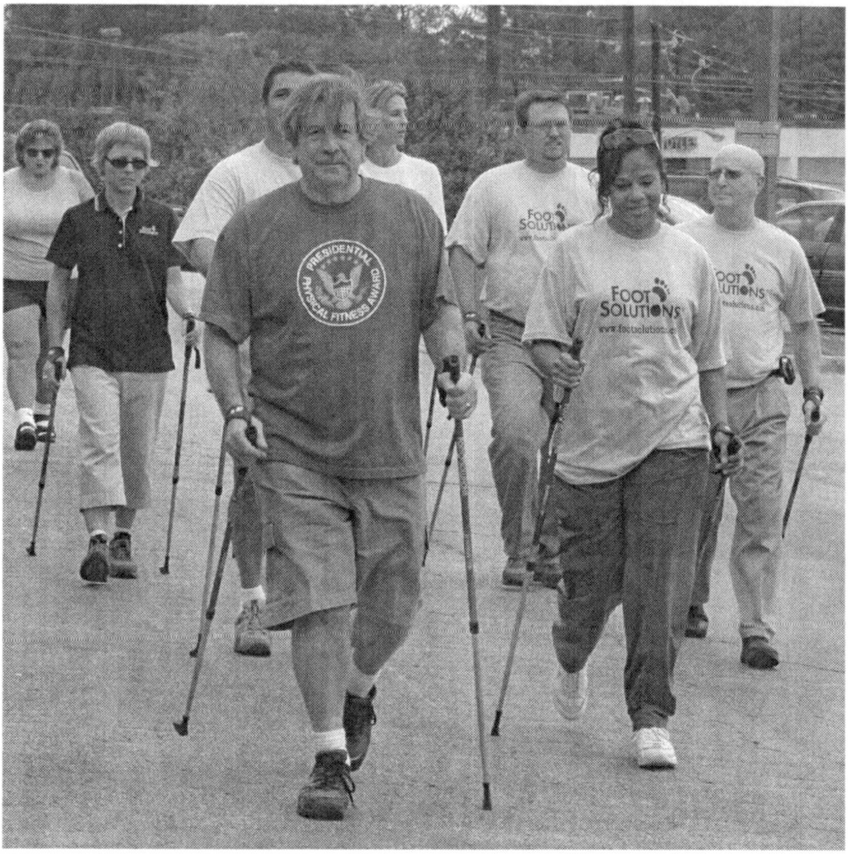


Join others across the world as they pledge to start a healthier BALANCED lifestyle.

Balance Walking is about creating balance in your life with some basic lifestyle changes that are easy to adapt to, making you look years younger and in turn produce a feeling of well being, fitness, strength and good health for the rest of your life. This simple system and approach will only take 15 minutes per day.

The core of the Balance Walking Way is based on Nordic Pole Walking using a specially designed Chung Shi shoe that helps accelerate the benefits of Pole Walking while also improving your body alignment and muscle tone. You will engage your core muscle groups while improving your balance and physical well being.

The Balance Walking Program covers four areas that are critical to improve the balance in ones life:

- Pole/Chung Shi walking for fitness
- Stress management and relaxation
- Strengthening and toning of your body
- Stimulate eating for pleasure and health

# Balance Walking Program with Chung Shi Shoes

It all starts with a uniquely designed shoe that will help accelerate your program. In addition you can wear this shoe all day for your normal activity, increasing the benefits without changing your schedule.

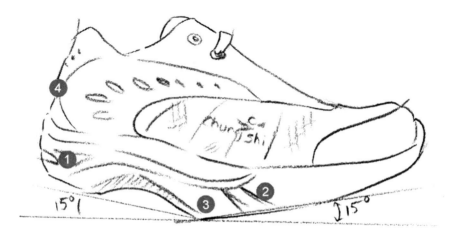


Feel more fit, more energized and motivated.

Keep going with Chung Shi!

Balance Walking

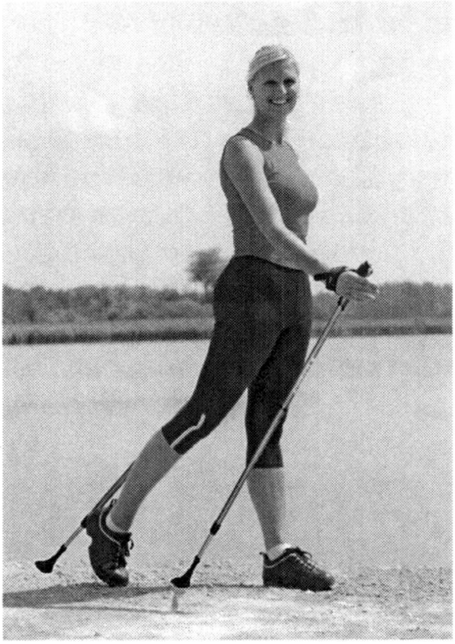

Whether you are wearing Chung Shi at the gym, Balance Walking, jogging or simply performing your everyday activities, your body will see increased toning, strengthened muscles, increased circulation and improved posture. You will feel fit and more energized with an overall improved sense of health and well-being. Natural, relaxed and upright movement is extremely comfortable for the entire body! Chung Shi allows you to stand, walk and jog in a more aligned position, making the neck, back, joints and feet comfortable. Better alignment challenges our core strengthening muscles to be more active, burning more calories and create a stronger, more toned and more stable body that is less prone to injury. Chung Shi reduces shock to the entire skeletal system at every step, making you feel better and motivated to keep moving.

## The secret is in the sole!

Chung Shi's unique, patented, angled sole encourages a soft heel strike with a natural, forward rolling action. Chung Shi directs the entire body to move through the proper biomechanical motion into a stable, correct gait with a shortened stride. The jarring action of walking and jogging on hard surfaces is greatly reduced. When standing, Chung Shi automatically puts the body into an aligned position, taking pressure off the neck, back, joints and feet. It's a better environment for the entire body.

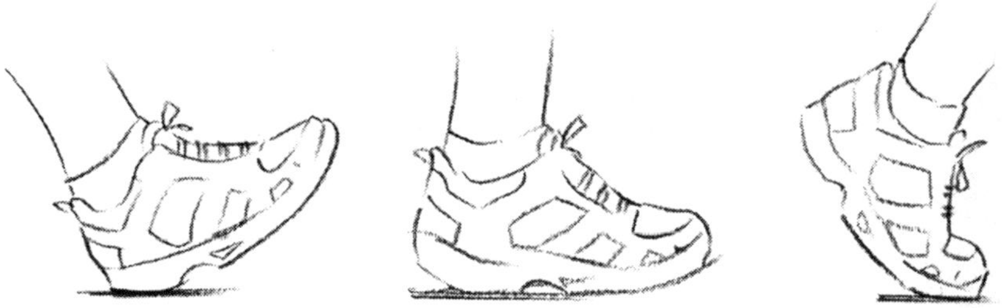

A B C

A) Angled sole aligns the body when standing and softens the heel strike, reducing jarring effect while walking or jogging.

B) The rolling ramp directs correct motion, promoting forward drive.

C) Angled sole directs a natural, propulsive rolling motion at toe-off that promotes an aligned gait.

Choose the level that's right for your body and your goals!

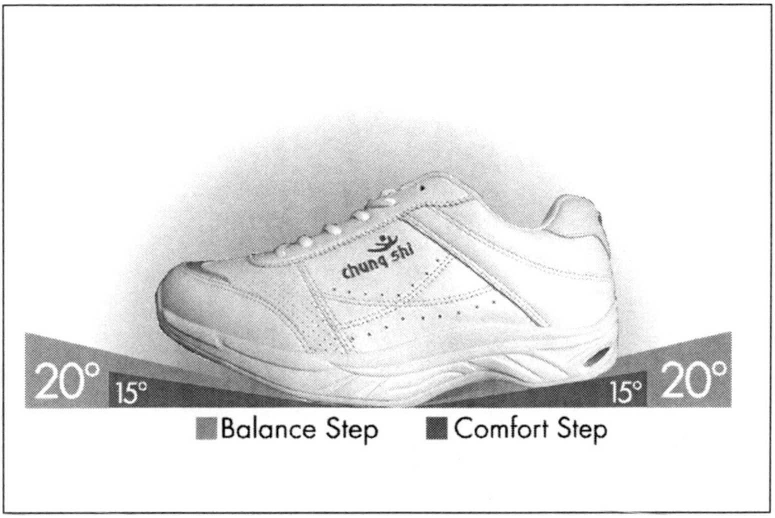


Chung Shi Comfort Step has a 15-degree angle at the heel and toe, creating a natural rolling motion that is perfect for standing, walking and jogging.

Chung Shi Balance Step takes your workout to an entirely new level. It features a 20-degree angle at the heel and toe and has a higher apex at the rolling ramp. This forces muscles to work much harder than Comfort Step. It is the most aggressive alignment and muscle-use shoe available.

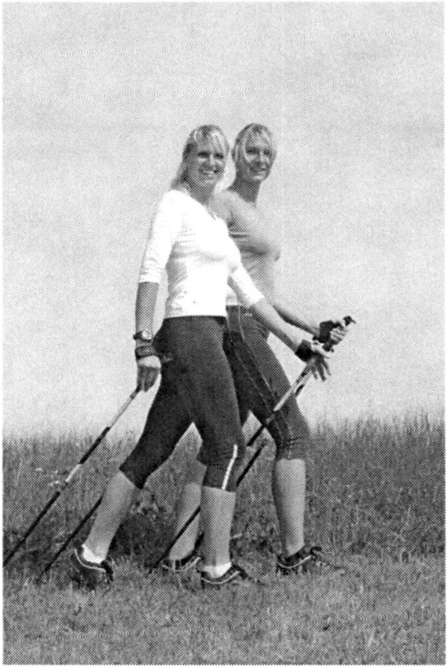

## Technical specification

Construction and classification of Chung Shi

Chung Shi meets the requirements of European guidelines for medical products and is rated a Class 1 Medical Device in Germany. The softening effect of Chung Shi is progressive, and provides the wearer with the correct amount of feedback from the walking surface (i.e. concrete, wood floors, turf, etc.) so that the body can adapt accordingly. This is important because much softening and shock absorption material in footwear creates instability, as well as inadequate feedback. Instability makes it more difficult to have correct posture, and can cause overuse of certain muscles and tendons, increasing the risk of injury.

The functionality of Chung Shi is based upon:

- A 15-degree (Comfort Step) or 20-degree (Balance Step) angle at the toe and heel of the shoe.
- The sole construction features a rolling ramp to direct the natural, forward-rolling, propulsive motion.

1. Stabilizer: An ergonomically shaped, stainless steel plate, which is both stabilizing and activating.

2. It is surrounded by a Polyurethane middle sole.

3. The rolling ramp in the middle promotes forward drive.

4. The heel is surrounded by a firm protective layer which stabilizes the entire foot.

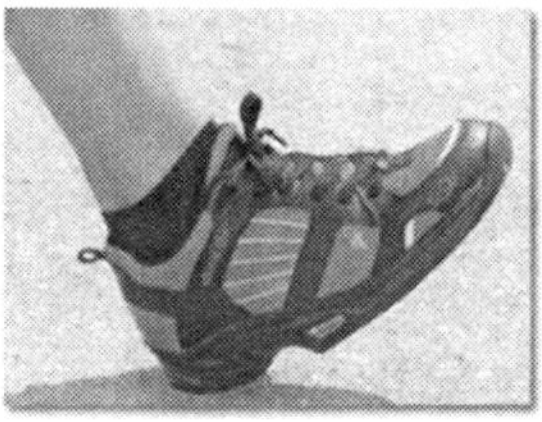

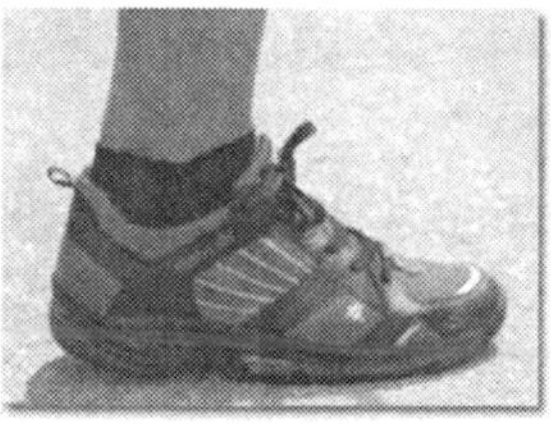

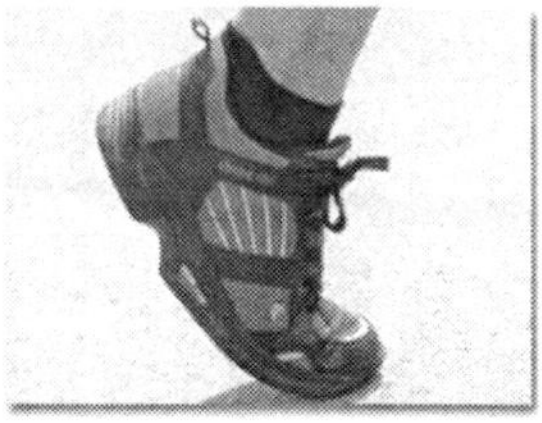

Benefits of Chung Shi Shoes

Health:

- Promotes the natural walking and jogging gait
- Achieves better postural alignment
- Absorbs shock to the feet, knees, hips and back
- Strengthens the core muscles
- Improves posture and relieves pressure on the vertebral column
- Increases circulation in the feet and legs
- Strengthens the muscles that support the pelvic floor
- Improves respiration
- Reduces overuse of tendons, ligaments and muscles
- Promotes a stronger, more resilient body, less prone to injury
- Activates the foot reflexology zones

Beauty:

- Increases calorie consumption (compared with "normal" shoes)
- Improves respiratory and circulatory function, strengthens and improves control of muscles leading to greater relaxation
- Finger-pressure massage effect of Chung Shi activates the reflexology zones of the feet
- Improved posture and gait leads to a more natural, relaxed stance and walking and running gait

- May improve or reduce varicose veins
- Improves the appearance of cellulite

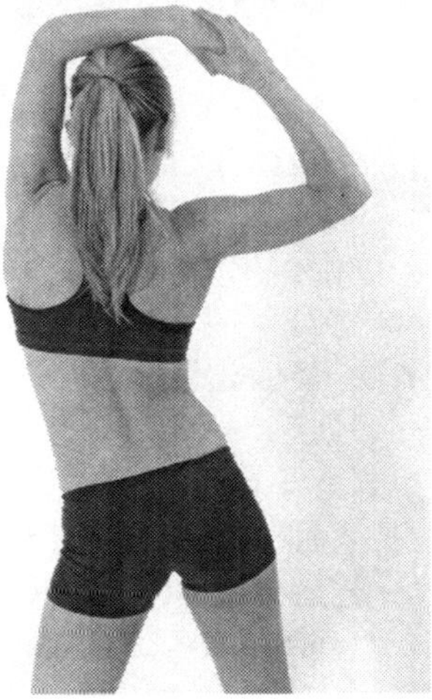

Fitness:

- Increases core stability
- Activates neglected muscles
- Improves athletic endurance
- Tones and strengthens the feet, legs, buttocks, abs and back
- Helps prevent injuries to tendons, ligaments and muscles
- Makes muscles work harder and, therefore, burn more calories
- Leads to a more relaxed, upright posture improving respiration

## Walking as nature intended

Chung Shi replicates the gait pattern and alignment of standing, walking and jogging on natural surfaces - the environment in which human beings have lived for thousands of years. The paved surfaces of modern life are convenient in many ways. However, they cause us to stand, walk and run differently, often causing our bodies to work in a misaligned position, creating foot, joint, back and even neck problems. Chung Shi gets you back to the aligned position that allows your body to work optimally.

## Strengthen and tone muscles

With the use of Chung Shi, neglected, underdeveloped muscles are activated. Chung Shi puts the body in better alignment, building core strength and stability. The muscles of the abs, buttocks, back, legs and feet are toned and strengthened. Chung Shi is an excellent training shoe, as it builds a stronger, more stable body that is more resilient and less prone to injury. And, Chung Shi targets and strengthens the pelvic floor muscles that weaken with age and pregnancy.

Better circulation means better health and better veins! Chung Shi increases muscle activity, generating an increased "blood pump" action. This helps to return blood from the extremities of the legs and feet back into the heart. Better circulation means reduced problems with varicose veins.

Enjoy a massage with every step! The rolling ramp in the middle of Chung Shi firmly touches the arch of the foot during walking and jogging producing a finger pressure massage which activates foot reflexology zones.

Relief for back and joint problems! Chung Shi alleviates numerous orthopedic and medical issues. The unique, patented sole directs the entire body through a more stable, less jarring, natural gait, improving total body alignment. The result is a decrease in joint pressure and a reduction of impact forces, and repeated muscular-skeletal compression at heel strike. Every time your heel strikes the ground, the impact to the heel is 3 to 5 times your body. Wearing Chung Shi reduces overuse of tendons, ligaments and muscles, and improves circulation, respiration and the biomechanical function of the entire body. Chung Shi helps the spinal column to return to a natural, relaxed and upright position, and is used by medical professionals to successfully prevent and treat a variety of conditions and injuries.

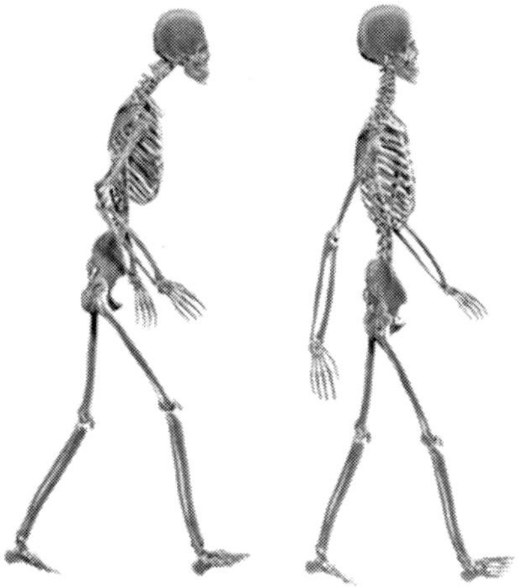

*Before* *After*

"Chung Shi is footwear we have long needed. I have treated patients with a wide array of foot and gait disorders. I have never seen footwear designed to so perfectly direct the feet and the body through the correct biomechanical gait as Chung Shi. Chung Shi really will change the quality of life for so many who either wish to prevent problems or those in need of relief from painful conditions such as plantar fasciitis, metatarsalgia, Achilles tendonitis, various joint fusions, as well as the knee, hip and back disorders that trouble millions of us."
-W. Faddock, D.P.M. CPED

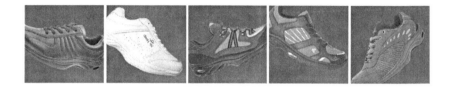

## East Meets West

A modern take on ancient wisdom

The foot is a complicated device designed to work best when on natural and uneven surfaces. Today's modern maze of hard flat surfaces, combined with poorly designed footwear, has created undue stress on our feet, knees, hips and back.

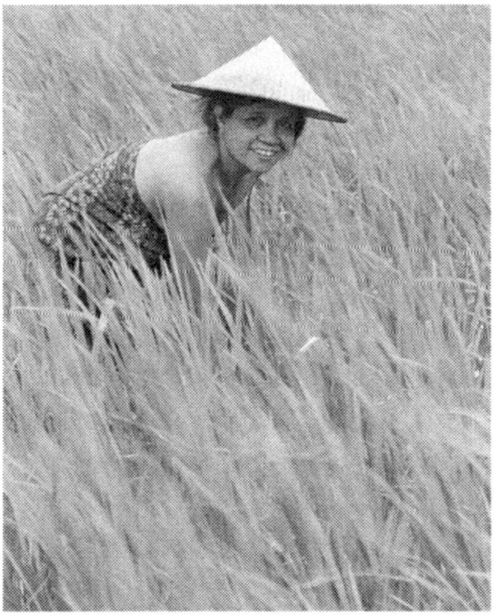

Go back in time

For thousands of years, Asians spent hours farming in rice paddies. They returned home to bamboo huts with bamboo floors and walkways. Walking on the uneven surfaces created a massage-like effect and roller action to the bottom of their feet, which helped to realign the entire body after a long day of bending over. As society evolved, even today, many Asians still walk on bamboo mats to relieve foot, leg and back issues.

Move forward

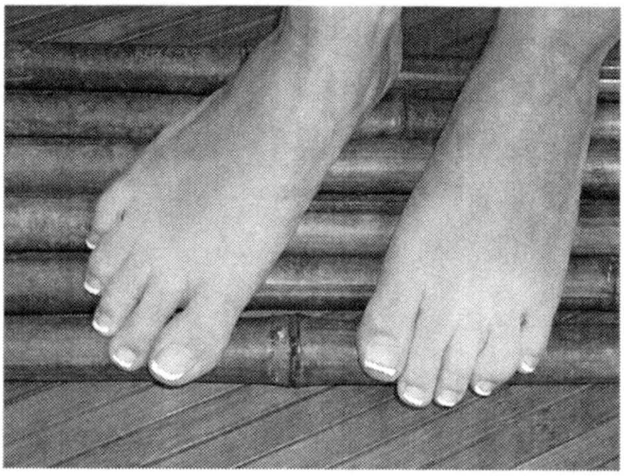

Learning from ancient Asian wisdom and adding modern German design and technology, the shoe for today is born. Chung Shi replaces the uneven bamboo mat with a patented sole, providing a massaging effect while walking or standing. This unique heel/toe design, combined with a center roll bar, supports the foot in a unique way that improves body alignment while reducing stress and shock to the spine.

Combining Chung Shi shoes and Nordic Pole Walking is the BASE FOUNDATION for the Balance Walking Program. Foot Solutions has several other exclusive footwear products that can also be used in conjunction with the Balance Walking program.

## Busy Lifestyles – Great Solution

Daily exercise, an essential component for good health, is fun and easy with FOOT SOLUTIONS Nordic Walking Poles. Double your benefits in just half the time.

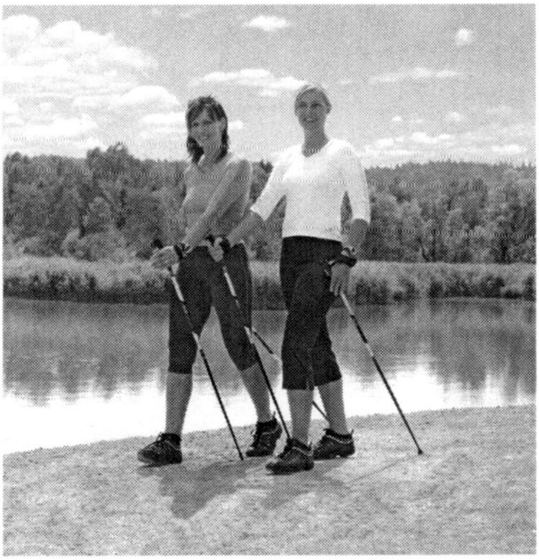

## More Benefits Than You Would Expect

Research and studies document the results. Thousands of individuals have made positive improvements in:

- Osteoporosis
- Obesity
- Diabetes
- Fibromyalgia
- Arthritis
- Pre post-natal care
- Surgery recovery
- Athletic training
- Depression
- And much more!

## Fitness Trend for the New Millennium

Nordic Pole Walking – the activity for anyone, anywhere, at any age, with any lifestyle. Nordic Pole Walking is inexpensive. Learn how now and walk with our well-established network of coaches and classes.

## Anyone Can Do This:

Age is not a barrier. The poles improve balance and stability making you more confident, as you continue to strengthen and tone. Feel fit and fabulous while you walk. Nordic Pole Walking is the fountain of youth we've all been searching for.

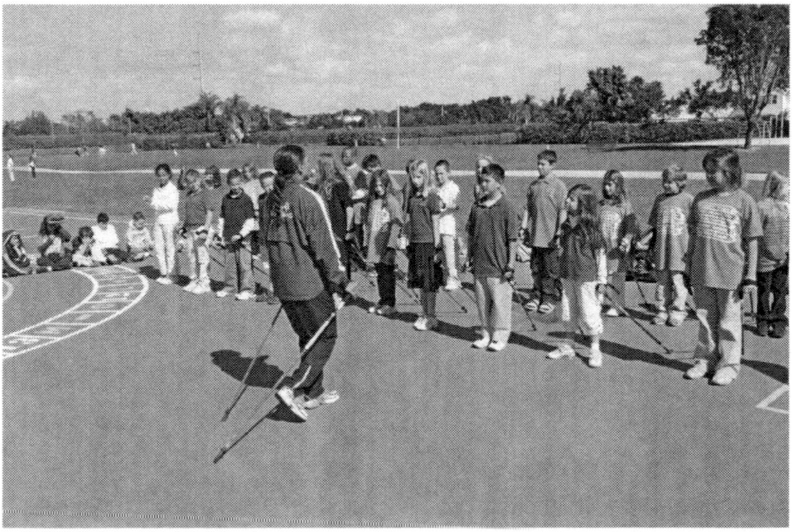

Children love Nordic pole walking too. They can walk, run, jump and train simply and safely, making this sporting activity a family affair that can bridge the generation gap.

Are you out of shape or inactive? No problem. Balance walking is truly a low-impact activity that is enjoyed by all fitness levels. From the couch potato to the elite athlete in training, Nordic Pole Walking from Foot Solutions will help get you into the best condition of your life.

What are people saying about Nordic Pole Walking with Foot Solutions Walk Clubs?

"My lifestyle is busy, and my body was unfortunately showing signs of inactivity and weight gain. My lower back was making it difficult to enjoy my students and family. I joined the Walk Club at school with my faculty friends and within the first 2 weeks my back pain WAS GONE and I had already lost 4 pounds."

-Robin T. – 2nd Grade Teacher & Mom

"As a 60-year-old active physician, it was immediately obvious the value of Nordic Pole Walking. Many of my patients were stuck in a rut of needing to exercise but not feeling comfortable in traditional gyms or training regimens. Nordic Pole Walking is the best low-impact, cardio activity I have come across. Our patients walk for their heart, their health and their life."

-Dr. Art L. – Heart Surgeon Inner City Hospital

"Our neighborhood Nordic Walking class has gotten the whole family outdoors together at least 3 times per week. We have significantly impacted our insulin dependence, improved family dynamics and feel great. There is even a high school program to get the teenagers on their feet whether they are track stars or in the marching band."'

-Michael, Michelle & Laura D.– A diabetic family

"Our busy practice has totally benefited from our FOOT SOLUTIONS Nordic Pole Walking Classes. We have pregnant moms, mature patients and staff, all walking, sharing ideas and staying fit. It's a win-win for women's health!"

-Nurse Denise M & Dr. Carol H – OB/GYN

"I'm a certified coach, retired U.S. Army Lieutenant Colonel, war vet, motivational speaker, an All-Army marathoner and track runner. I've run; I've coached; I've trained. Never before, have I encountered an activity that is perfect for elite athletes as a recovery and training tool and, at the same time, perfect for the majority of our population."

-Coach Sue B- a USATF, RRCA and Nordic Pole Walking Master instructor.

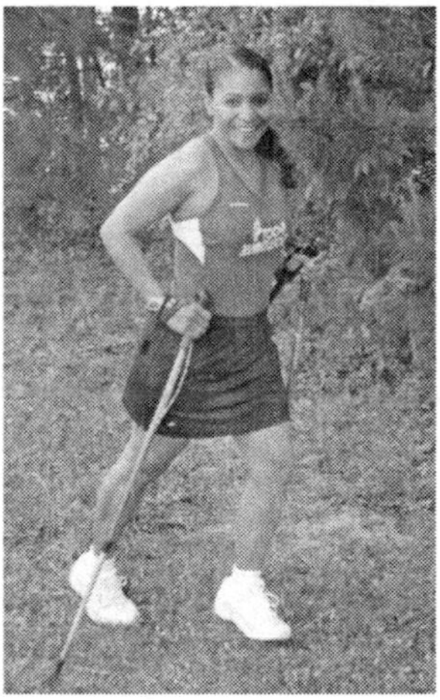

A number of elite runners are now using the Balance walking program as a low impact recovery method.

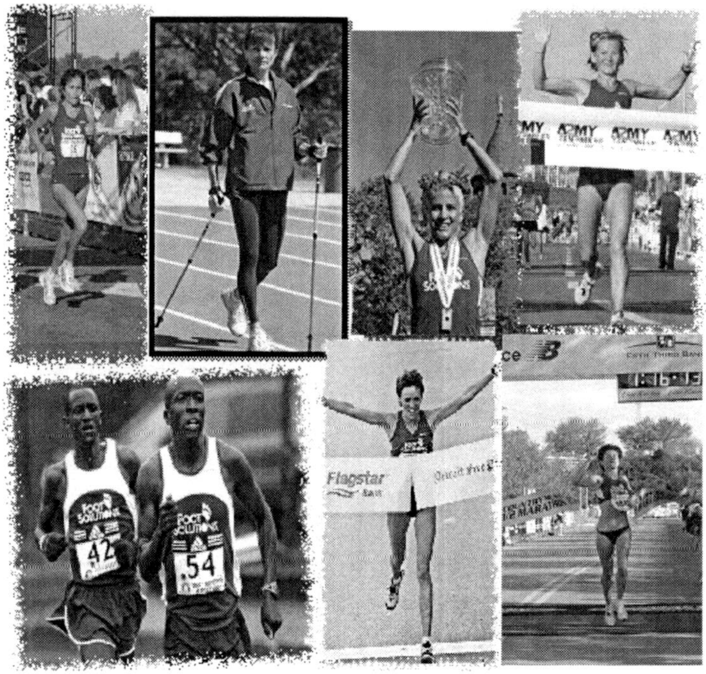

## Health & Wellness Benefits

The physical fitness part of Balance walking may be described as cross-country skiing without skis, exercises the entire body encouraging an upright posture and balance without placing unnecessary stress on the muscles, ligaments and tendons. Participants use modified ski poles and specially designed Chung Shi shoes.

Bottom line: Balance walking allows walkers to use their entire body while maintaining perfect posture and burning 50% more calories.

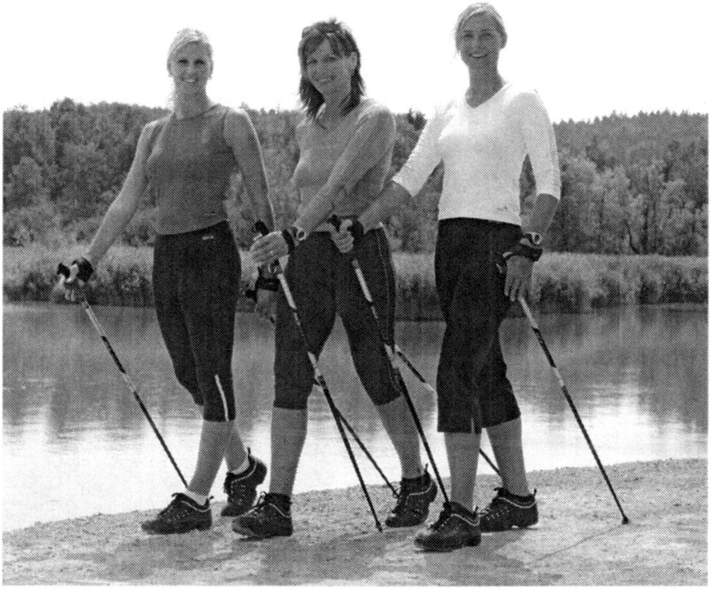

- Burns up to 46% more calories compared to traditional walking

- Cooper Institute, 2004

- Strengthens core muscles – toning abs, buttocks & back muscles
- Reduces stress to knees, hips & back up to 30%.

- Wilson, 2001

- Increases strength & endurance
- Enhances cardiovascular performance up to 22%

- Foley 1994

## A TOTAL BODY WORKOUT INCORPORATING UP TO 90% OF YOUR MUSCLES!

Visit www.balancewalking.com for detail information on a number of validation studies and reference information.

Half of the battle is to BELIEVE in yourself, the 2nd half, is the desire to do it.

"If you think you are beaten, you are; if you think you dare not, you don't; if you like to win but think you can't, it is almost certain you won't!

If you think you'll lose, you've lost; for in our world we find success begins with a person's will. It's all in the state of mind!

If you think you are outclassed, you are; you've got to think high to rise. You've got to be sure of yourself before you can even win the prize.

Life's battles don't always go to the stronger or the faster one, but sooner or later the one who wins is the one who thinks he or she can!" (Author of poem, unknown).

# Balance Walking & Weight Issues

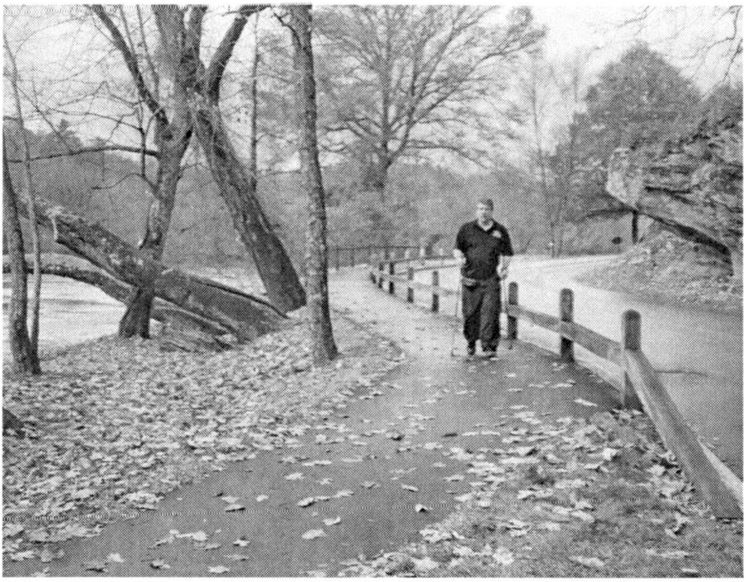

Just why does the world need one more exercise program when it seems every year there are a slew of new exercise programs, new fad diets, new miracle pills, new revolutionary equipment and gimmicks to help you lose weight, eliminate cellulite, find your six-pack (abs), etc., etc.? The problem is our world has become lazy and fat; our lifestyles are very different than they were just twenty-five years ago. Let's take a quick check on the state we are in.

Approximately two-thirds of U.S. adults are overweight, and one-third of the population is obese. Imagine that we are living in a time when one of every adult American weighs as much as the other two. Just twenty-five years ago, this number was less than 50% of what it is today.

This is not about how you look. It is about your health and life. The Surgeon General estimates well over $100 billion a year are spent on medical illnesses related to obesity and it is increasing every year. What are some of the side benefits of carrying that extra poundage? Heart disease, high blood pressure, stroke, diabetes, infertility, gall bladder disease, osteoarthritis and many types of cancer.

It is not just adults. The stage is already set for our children. Fifteen percent of U.S. children are obese, 15% overweight and another 20% borderline. Boy, do they have an unfortunate head start over our generation with their eating habits, lack of exercise, and addiction to television and electronic games.

Let's face it. We have created a "NOW SOCIETY." Everyone wants instant gratification and quick fixes, to his or her lives, whatever the problem or issue is. We are the richest nation in the world and the envy of the rest of the world, yet most of Americans are chronic complainers and do not appreciate the unbelievable luck they have had to have been born in America. Thanks to modern technology and mass production, food is not only readily available, but it is also inexpensive.

Balance Walking is about changing your lifestyle. The objective is to introduce more balance into you and your family's lives. This includes more quality time with your family, time for yourself to find some inner peace, eating in a more balanced way and introducing a moderate exercise plan that is efficient, simple and based on proven principles.

Some of the changes could be just reducing the amount of television, computer games, etc. that not only your children but you also spend time on. Finding and using wisely, just 15 to 30 minutes a day will change your life.

We are now looking for a more balanced lifestyle, not only with what we eat, but also with increasing our level of physical activity using Balance Walking as the basis for this increase. Most of us are already in trouble because of our environment – fast and convenient food with oversized portions. It's not about quality any longer; instead, it's about quantity. Americans are among the hardest working people in the world yet most of us are stressed and have little to no personal time. We also suffer from information overload. Add to this our lack of time and level of inactivity; they all contribute to our own demise.

I apologize for getting a little philosophical and negative here, but look around for yourself. Many of us just need to take an honest look in the mirror; this is really my major reason for writing this book. I have looked in the mirror and I didn't like who was staring back at me. I am a workaholic and operate on 5 hours of sleep on average per night. Life has been good to me – I live a very active lifestyle and at 55 years of age I was the same weight as I was at 21 and still had a 32" waist. Then things changed and all of a sudden I was adding about five pounds per year. This small gain has a way of sneaking up on you. Now I am looking at a person 40 pounds heavier and easily a 38" waist. This is my wake up call and Balance Walking is the result of my research on how to live a more balanced lifestyle and make changes I can live with. The amount of time it requires to make changes to your life was a very important component of establishing this program. Let me emphasize Balance Walking is NOT focused on getting you to look like a movie star (but it could) or about dieting and forcing you into a self-defeating way of life. It is about bringing balance into your life and helping you find the best way for you to enjoy your journey through life. It is about changing your lifestyle for the rest of your life with several simple steps that are very easy to accomplish.

It's about living a full, active lifestyle for your complete life, not just part of it. THIS IS ABOUT YOU!

**Enjoy the journey, after all, that is what life is all about.**

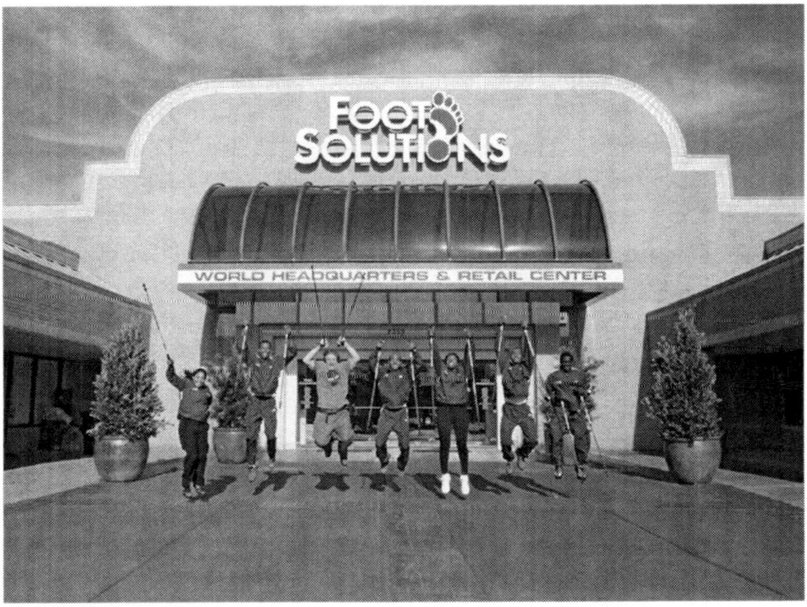


Ray & the Foot Solutions running team celebrating the moment.

Time – our most precious commodity yet most of us do not use it wisely

The Balance Walking Way allows you to change your lifestyle and with as little as 15 minutes per day you will start to notice a difference within weeks! This is a low-impact, low-stress way to exercise 90% of your muscles and get up to a 50% increase in calories burned over regular walking.

Balance Walking can help you live a longer, healthier, more active life. It can literally stop the clock of time for some and turn it back for others. There is no magic fountain of youth, but nature has provided simple solutions to help you live a much happier, fuller life without taking extreme measures. This process is about enjoying life but also using some of your time effectively.

## What are the basic needs for life?

Oxygen, water, nutrition, exercise and rest; pretty basic and simple. So, why do we have to make life so difficult and complex? Even more distressing, the World Health Organization rates every country's health. Japan is on top of the list for the healthiest country in the world while, to my surprise, the United States was well down the list. Unbelievably, there are over forty countries ranked as being healthier than the United States. How can this be when the United States has the most advanced and finest healthcare facilities in the world, as well as some of the most expensive? Yet here we are ranked right at the top of the list for heart disease, cancer, diabetes, arthritis and obesity, which is a major contributor to the health of our country. There is no question that our lifestyles and diets have a lot to do with this.

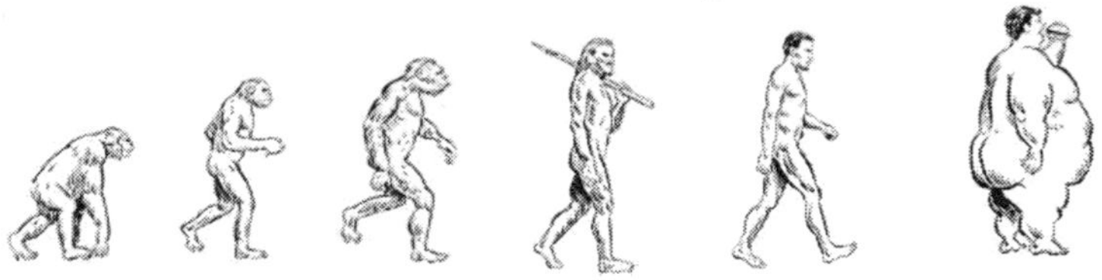

Yet we fail to get the message even though this has been documented over and over again in medical journals, countless magazine articles and now even TV specials and news channels. Look around you; weight loss diets, gimmicks and pills are a multi billion dollar industry, yet we continue to get heavier. The fix is really simple and has always been available to you. Balance Walking can help you change your lifestyle because that is the issue on the table; there are no quick fixes that work; over time most people regain their weight loss plus. You must choose to change your lifestyle for the rest of your life if you want change and success. Before you assume that this is just another gimmick or diet, please read on; Balance Walking uses proven concepts and principles that are natural and, just as its name suggests, is about putting balance in your life. First, you must accept that you want change in your life; then you have to take responsibility for yourself and your life. You must consider preventative maintenance instead of thinking that traditional medicine and surgery are the only solutions. You must consider lifestyle changes that become part of your life for the rest of your life. Obviously if you have medical problems or issues you must use traditional medical solutions. This is about doing something for your self before there is a problem. However, the body can do remarkable things to heal itself and there are many studies done in Germany and other European countries on specific disease-related issues and Nordic Pole Walking.

Let's start with some simple changes like eating healthier, think about quality and freshness, not quantity. I am not suggesting going on a diet, we should ban the word diet. It doesn't work because it is not natural. Let's face it; having to trick your body and punish yourself is not a long term solution and has not worked in the past. Also, we don't need another study on why we are getting fat. Why do you think you are gaining or shifting weight? Yes, it's pretty simple, isn't it? We can see that dieting does not work with the number of alternate programs, fads and businesses that advertise weight loss solutions. If any of these solutions really worked and had long lasting results, there would not be a new fad diet on the bestseller list every year or countless other alternative solutions and we would be winning the battle of the bulge instead of losing it!

Let's face it. The more you are told not to eat something, the more you want it! Keep it simple. Do not ride the roller coaster of food and sugar intake. Did you know the average American consumes approximately 3 pounds of sugar per week? You are not a wild animal that does not know when its next meal will come. Eat simple, four to six smaller meals everyday. Eat what you want if you have the urge, but take smaller portions and enjoy the taste and the moment. Eat slowly; taste each bite and satisfy the urge and the craving. It's not about how much you can shove into your furnace; it's really about how much you can burn. However, whenever you can, try to make the healthier choice. It really is that simple. Look at the French or the Italians. Eating is an important part of life and also one of the most enjoyable. Both countries have wonderful dishes with no restraint. They use natural, fresh products and stay away from processed foods and heavy use of sugar; their portions are very reasonable in size. That is the one hurdle you must get over – food is a celebration of life. Enjoy it! I have recently spent time in Germany, Holland and Italy. Since

I am conscientious about the issues we face in the U.S., I could not help but notice the difference between us. Although I am sure they exist everywhere, I did not see one really obese person on the trip and had to really search just to find some overweight people. Even middle-aged and older people were in such better physical shape and appearance than in the U.S. It is very simple to see that just small changes in the way people live and eat support what we already know.

Through the combination of several elements, including Balance Walking, relaxation, basic flexibility, muscle toning and a practical approach to eating (NOT DIETING), the Balance Walking Way will allow you to change your lifestyle and do more in less time with increased benefits! You can change your life with as little as 15 minutes per day. If you can dedicate 30 minutes you will get even more results, but start with very achievable commitments; 15 minutes may be all you need or can afford at this time.

This program is for anyone at any age - young or old - and is designed to be right for your individual needs. Simply put, you decide and define what you want to accomplish and how much time you want to dedicate. Balance Walking is designed to accommodate your busy lifestyle without major change. It can be done anywhere, anytime, and during any season. Balance Walking is a way of life designed to put your life in balance. This very simplistic approach is all that is needed and it will certainly change your life and the way you feel, look and act. Are you ready to turn back the clock and kick start your energy level?

Balance Walking can help you whether you are just getting started with simple goals or if you are an elite athlete. Balance Walking is even effective for children who need to be entertained, as well as for the elderly that will feel more confident because the walking poles give them more stability while still allowing them to be active. We have seen this firsthand when our coaches have visited retirement groups for presentations and offered free lessons on Balance Walking as well as with children in schools.

What if we could reverse the aging process, stop time and literally look and feel ten years younger or more? People spend millions of dollars every year trying to do just that. Just think about it for a moment. Money is spent on everything from plastic surgery, liposuction, and tummy tucks to diet pills, magic formulas, and even creams promising to build muscle, diminish fat and make cellulite disappear. Everyone wants the easy way out. How many of us have the time, willpower or desire to spend hours every day in the gym trying to hone our bodies to perfection? Most of us have to work and have a life to live. Some of us are in such bad shape it is a struggle just to walk upstairs, and easily over one-third of us just flat out have to change our lifestyles now if we want to avoid serious issues in the very near future.

## Posture & Body Alignment

What is it that you do and don't want out of life? Do you want a body that can take you there? What about for your children?

Today, it's easy to see that the apple did not fall too far from the tree; look at an overweight parent and most likely you will see an overweight child. Please don't assume it is all about bad genes. It is true that a very small percentage of people do have a medical issue or some genetic problem, but the chances are so small that it is not an acceptable excuse for you, unless you really do have a medical problem.

Let's discuss what makes you look and feel younger. Let's start with posture.

**POSTURE** – if you are standing in correct body alignment, what happens? You are taller, you breathe easier, you look slimmer, and you eliminate aches and pains in the feet, knees, hip, back and neck. This is true because if your body is in the correct body alignment, your weight distribution is evened out and many muscles and ligaments do not have to strain to help adjust for body misalignment. Yet, most of us sit and stand incorrectly. If you visit a chiropractor, what does the doctor do? In my experience he or she starts with my feet and begins lining up my body through a series of adjustments, all the way up to my neck with that last quick neck adjustment that always makes me cringe, but feels good. If you can maintain that, correct adjustment and posture, many aches and pains will disappear. I have been hunched over a desk and computer for years, but by just wearing my Chung Shi shoes every day at work people began noticing that I looked different. My body alignment changed just because of this specialty shoe. I personally noticed the difference immediately when I first tried them on.

Balance Walking will give you a noted improvement in posture and body alignment. This is part of the basic program and can be accomplished all day, just by wearing these specially designed Chung Shi shoes. This is one element alone that can substantially reduce pain issues in your feet, knees, hips, back and neck.

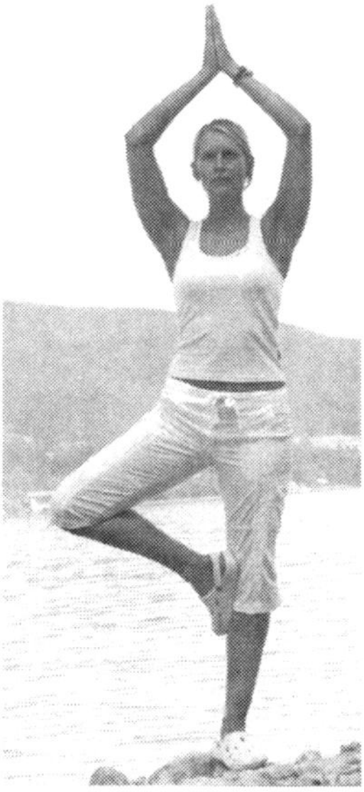

**FLEXIBILITY** – As we age, because of lack of use and proper stretching, our muscles, ligaments and tendons lose some of their shape, form and elasticity. Many of us can no longer bend over easily to tie our shoelaces. We have to kneel or sit, yet most of us could easily touch the floor when we were younger. In fact, this is another area that reflects on how we look and how old we feel. Yet, look at older people that practice yoga or tai chi. They maintain their flexibility and their movements are very fluid. In fact, many older people that practice yoga can easily put their palms on the floor by simply bending over. The greatest thing about the body is that it will heal and help itself if you help it, you can see remarkable changes in your body and flexibility. It is not too late to start today no matter how old you are.

**ENDURANCE** – Use it or lose it! This definitely applies to the body, which is a complex engineering marvel. I am not talking about running marathons, although there are many senior citizens doing just that. Let's talk basics. How about just walking from the car to the mall at a brisk pace? I grew up in New England and every winter there was another neighbor suffering a heart attack while shoveling snow. How does this happen? Very simply; you cannot lay around watching television and stuffing your body with all the wrong foods then go out and shovel the driveway without some consequences. Ask anyone that has shoveled a driveway, it is serious work; if you are out of shape you will strain yourself and there will be consequences. Endurance is important because it allows us to stay more active and enjoy life to the fullest. It wasn't too many generations ago when you survived by a decision of flight or fight. Endurance then could mean the difference between life and death. We may not still be living in the jungle, but many daily events could require us to move a little faster or require a little endurance that could save our life. How about just playing with your children or grandchildren, I mean really playing; or going out to shovel snow from the driveway.

**TONE & SHAPE** – Having muscle tone and shape is certainly high on the list if you want to look and feel younger. Most people, as they age, have let themselves go and most of their muscle has turned to what? Do I have to say it? Look in the mirror. I mean really look. You have gotten used to the person looking back at you over the years. Furthermore you have accepted and adjusted to who you are and what you have become, and the person looking back at you is you. By the way, no one else is seeing you the same way you see yourself. When was the last time you were at the beach and saw a person in a swimsuit or an outfit at a dinner party that had you asking yourself, "what could that person have been thinking?" Maybe you are that person. It is hard to accept that our bodies are changing, but once they start, it is like a dam giving way and the rampage does not stop. It could be as simple as five pounds per year. In five years, that's twenty-five pounds.

What about muscle mass? Most people start losing muscle mass at age 30. Want the simple truth? Pull a picture of yourself out of your scrapbook from ten years ago. Did you look different? If not, go deeper into the scrapbook. I want you looking at the body you once had. It is still inside of you, just hidden under a few layers. I did this with my daughter, who is 6-years old. The picture was only about ten years ago. Her comment to me was "You look different, why is your tummy so big!" and she was right. I looked about forty pounds different, tough to accept when your children have to bring you back to reality. Tone and shape are definitely on the list if you want a change in your life. Maintaining muscle mass and bone density are critical factors as we age. Women and men have different toning issues and areas, and we will address both.

Did you know that falling is the third leading cause of death for the elderly? Improved balance, agility, muscle control and increased bone density will all reduce this statistic and could keep you alive longer.

**WEIGHT CONTROL** - Where do I start? Out-of-control weight is not healthy. It's a major contributor to diabetes, heart problems and a slew of other problems. Yet, here we are, in a country where one person out of three people weighs as much as the other two combined. Weight management is out of control not only for the elderly, but for the middle-aged as well. Now, even our children are dealing with obesity. Our highly processed foods, lack of exercise and diminished quality of life are leading us to extinction. This is probably the number one problem and issue for many of you, and I know you have probably tried many things unsuccessfully. Let's not focus on this issue now, but I promise you results if you try the Balance Walking Program for just thirty days. The thirty days are hopefully just what you need to whet your appetite. We want this to be a lifestyle change. If you do not see or notice a change in yourself please email me, and I will personally refund to you the cost of this book.

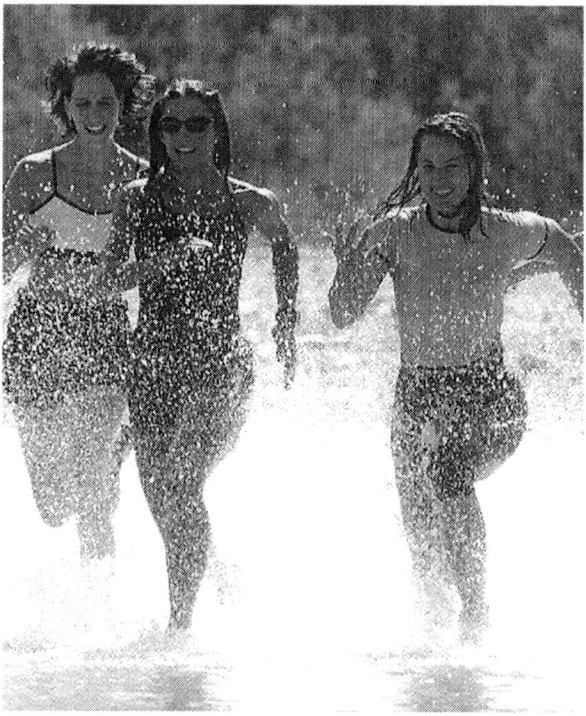

**ENERGY** – People that look and feel younger just seem to have more energy... more zest for life. If you are a baby boomer, you want more out of life and you are not ready for the rocking chair on the porch just yet. In fact, the Baby Boomer wants to live a lifestyle that defies age and gravity and will do anything to achieve this. I agree that energy is like the fountain of youth and there is absolutely no reason why you cannot get an adrenaline rush and boost your energy levels the natural way. Energy will come to you with the Balance Walking Way.

**LIFESTYLE** – This means many things to each of us. The bottom line is that you want to change your life. You don't know why, but you are ready for change. Let's start by not blaming anyone or anything for where we are right now. Implement and follow the Balance Walking Way for you. That is right. This is all about you! You may encourage family and friends to look into Balance Walking. It is always easier to change one's lifestyle with a support group. However, no matter what, stay focused! This is all about you and the rest of your life. Remember you cannot change a person that does not want to change. Do not blame your spouse, your job, your parents or anyone else for why you are where you are. Just simply decide that you are going to help yourself; do not become fanatical. We are talking about simpler lifestyle changes that will have a substantial impact on you. In America everything is all about extremes and quick fixes. Unfortunately this is what we want to change, we are talking about small, incremental changes that are easy to adjust to and live with. Let's think turtle; we want to finish the race.

The objective of the Balance Walking Way is to put balance back in your life. We will borrow from a number of different disciplines from simple, proven sources that have survived the test of time and combine them into simple lifestyle changes that will allow you to get results in a time frame that is right for you. Remember, we are talking about lifestyle changes that, to some degree, you will do for the rest of your life. Do this in bite-size chunks that work for you. You are not competing with anyone. This is all about inner satisfaction and peace with oneself.

# Cornerstone of Balance Walking - Nordic Pole Walking

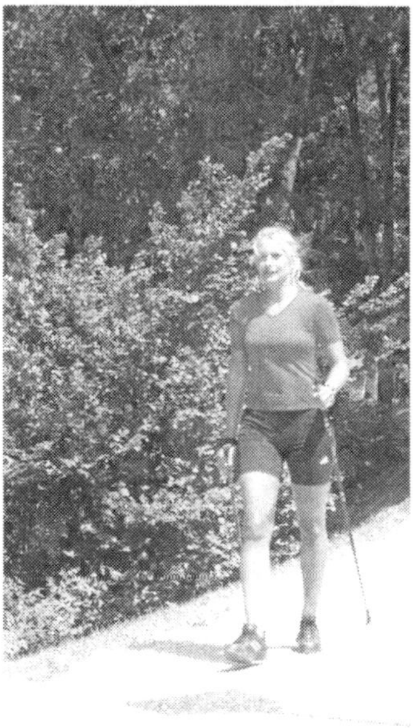

Let's start with the foundation of the Balance Walking Way. The physical and aerobic portion is based primarily on Nordic Pole Walking using a specially designed shoe available only at Foot Solutions to increase the results of your walking program in less time. That's right, this combination will increase your calorie burn rate by 50% over regular walking; you will see results with only 15 minutes a day.

As a young man in upstate New York, I used to cross-country ski on the trails.

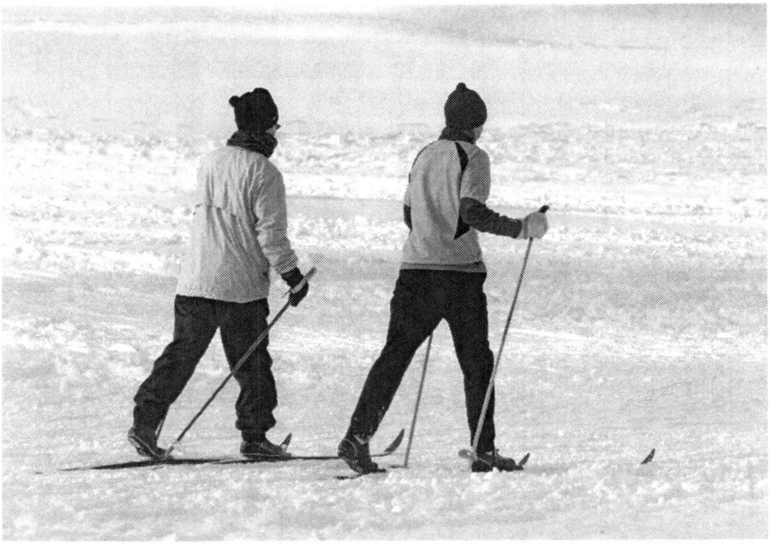

We will not be cross-country skiing, so don't get too excited; we will be using the concept of pole walking with a specially designed Chung Shi Balance Walking shoe for the physical and endurance part of this program. You can make it as simple and relaxing as you want or, you can push yourself to the limit.

Pole walking has been well documented over the years and there are hundreds of validated studies. It has been the most successful in Finland and Germany in recent years with even medical insurance companies substantiating the unbelievably positive results and offering major reductions in healthcare costs.

Being an entrepreneur and visionary, I cannot leave anything alone. I always have to take something and improve on it. It is my nature and what I do best. Since I have been exposed to so many parts of the world and their cultures, diets and lifestyles, I see Balance walking as a combination of what I learned on those travels and a lifetime of research, testing and experimenting. In actuality, all the parts of the puzzle have existed for many years. This is just a simple combination of components that make sense and are already well proven independently, but combined, they are a very effective way to impact your life today with minimal time, less strain and maximal benefits.

## IT ALL STARTS WITH THE FEET

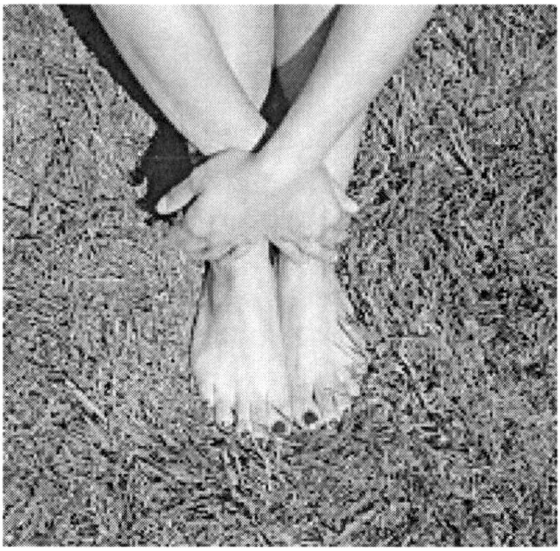

The human foot contains 26 bones, 33 joints and over 100 tendons, muscles and ligament.

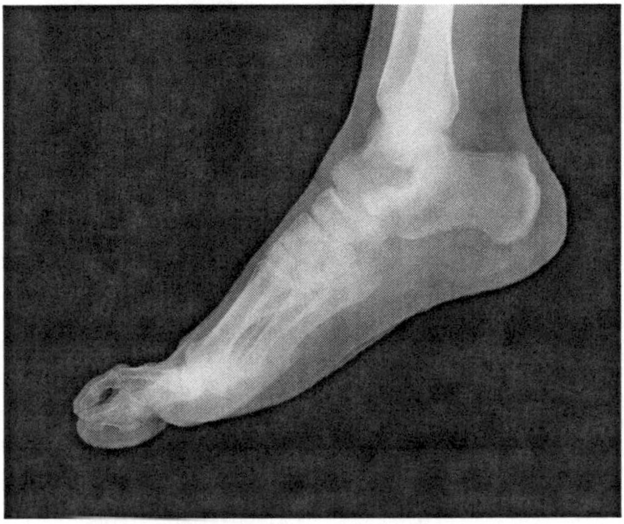

Taking care of your feet is taking care of the whole you. Did you know that the average person walks the equivalent of 3.5 times around the world during his or her lifetime?

The human foot contains twenty-six bones, thirty-three joints and over one hundred tendons, muscles and ligaments. This is not only a very complicated part of our bodies, but it was designed to walk on uneven surfaces, not the flat concrete and hard surfaces man has created. In addition, ninety percent of all people wear improperly fitted shoes, which aggravate or cause the majority of foot pain and problems.

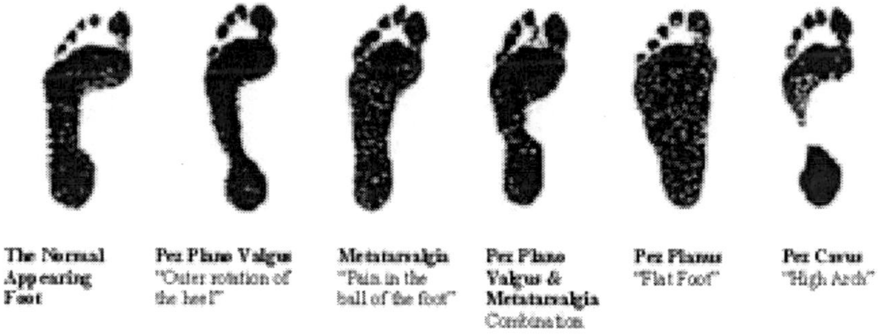


**Every foot is different, just like a snowflake.**

Feet come in all sizes and shapes, yet the majority of shoes are built to fit the masses. It is no wonder that what you wear on your feet is the most important part of foot care. Many problems such as aches in your feet, ankles, knees, lower back, and even your shoulders and neck, stem from improper support of your feet. A supportive shoe combined with a properly designed arch support will put your feet in their natural position for walking and standing, creating the correct foundation for your feet and the rest of your body. By putting your feet in balance, the alignment of other joints will be improved. Just ask your chiropractor about proper body alignment and what it means to you. If you have ever gone in for an adjustment, where does the chiropractor start? They begin with your feet. I was recently talking with a well-known neurosurgeon in Italy who told me that with many of his patients, he starts his assessment with the feet and proper body alignment.

While we are on the topic of discussing feet and support, I suggest you visit your nearest Foot Solutions store. Mention to the associate your interest in Balance Walking and you'll get a free computer foot-mapping analysis, gait analysis and foot-fitting analysis and assessment. This will take about twenty minutes, with a Foot Solutions professional trained in foot pathology and pedorthics. This analysis will give you a foot care plan for preventative maintenance, proper fit and support as well as solutions for actual foot problems and issues that you may have.

Our feet are the most complicated yet neglected parts of our bodies.

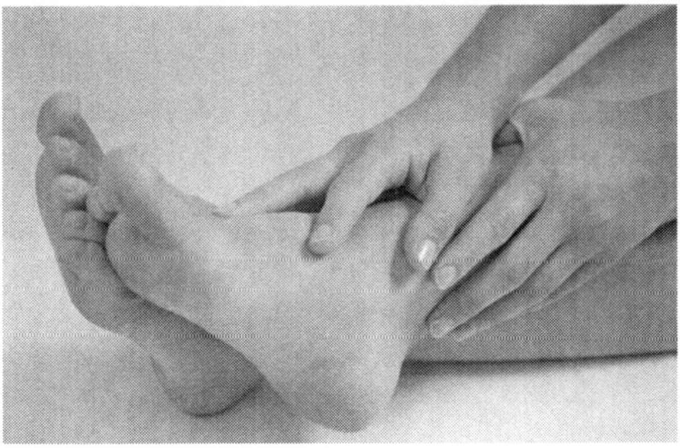

## What has all of this got to do with Balance Walking?

Balance Walking starts with your feet. Specially designed shoes and custom arch supports will change the way you stand and walk and are important factors for your long term success and well-being. Remember earlier, I mentioned that the feet are very complicated mechanical devices not designed for the flat, hard surfaces we live with and walk on daily.

For the full benefits of Balance Walking, I recommend the Chung Shi shoe. The Chung Shi shoe is a very unique shoe that will feel a bit odd at first, but once you wear them for several days, you will not want to take them off! These are some of the typical questions I get regarding Chung Shi shoes.

**Q:** What makes Chung Shi so special?

**A:** The angled sole of Chung Shi encourages a soft heel strike with a natural, forward-rolling action. Chung Shi directs the entire body to move through the proper biomechanical motion into a stable, correct gait with a shortened stride.

Chung Shi allows the body to walk in a naturally aligned posture (as you do on a natural, uneven surface such as wet sand) while on the paved surfaces of modern life. From a biomechanical perspective, walking in alignment allows the body to function most efficiently. This leads to better posture, increased muscle use, toning and strengthening of muscles in the feet, legs, buttocks, abs and back, reduced pressure on the back, joints and feet, improved circulation and respiration, increased calorie consumption, and a greater sense of health and well-being.

In alignment, pressure is taken off of the back and the joints, so those who suffer back and joint pain often feel significant relief. And, because of the unique, angled structure of the sole, pressure is moved away from the heel and ball of the foot, where most foot discomfort originates.

Additionally, Chung Shi builds underdeveloped muscles which increases muscle mass in the body and in turn helps burn more calories. And, because Chung Shi forces the muscles to move through a greater range of motion, there is greater calorie burn with every step. The increased range of motion also increases the "blood pump" effect, which improves circulation to the legs and feet.

Because Chung Shi encourages a more relaxed, upright posture that feels so good, you are more likely to remain motivated to exercise when wearing them.

Orthotics can be worn with Chung Shi, even in their sandals. Chung Shi is available in the following two levels. Chung Shi Comfort Step (Level One) has a 15 degree angle at the heel and toe, creating a natural, rolling motion that is perfect for every day use, standing, walking and jogging. Chung Shi Balance-Step (Level Two) takes your workout to an entirely new level. It features a 20 degree angle at the heel and toe and has a higher apex at the rolling ramp. This forces muscles to work much harder than the Comfort Step. It is the most aggressive alignment and muscle-use footwear available for the person that wants a greater challenge. I recommend the Balance Step 20 degree angled sole for your Balance Walking program. Another positive aspect in the design of this shoe is that it travels well. If you are on a plane a lot more than you would like and many flights are long, with your Chung Shi shoes, you can actually do flex exercises with your feet while sitting in your cramped seat. This simple flex exercise will actually increase the circulation of blood in your legs, a really important factor for frequent travelers.

**Q:** I just started a Nordic Pole Walking Program and I want to maximize my workout. Will Chung Shi help?

**A:** Yes. Because Chung Shi puts the body in a more aligned, upright posture, the muscles (which work in antagonistic pairs like a pulley system) are worked more evenly, building up the underworked muscles while alleviating the overworked muscles. This increases muscle mass in the body, which helps to burn more calories. Additionally because Chung Shi forces the muscles to move through a greater range of motion, more calories are burned with every step. This also increases flexibility, especially to the Achilles tendon. Chung Shi engages the core muscles, thereby building core stability.

Chung Shi is available in two levels, so you can choose the level appropriate to your fitness goals. The Level Two Balance Step takes all the key benefits of Level One Comfort Step to the maximum, working muscles harder while further increasing the circulation and massage-like effect with every step.

While your posture is aligned, your body is able to absorb the shock of each step more efficiently, reducing the chance of athletic injury. And, because Chung Shi encourages a more relaxed, upright posture that feels so good, you are more likely to remain motivated to exercise when wearing them.

**Q:** Can I jog while Balance Walking in Chung Shi shoes?

**A:** You are encouraged to jog in them, if you wish. However, just as in walking, the posture is one of alignment. This means you will be working muscles differently than when jogging in traditional shoes. It is strongly advised that you begin by walking in Chung Shi shoes first, and then gradually work up to jogging to avoid overuse of muscles that are not used to working in the aligned position.

Also, if you enjoy trail jogging or pole walking, Chung Shi is the perfect companion for the rugged, off-the-beaten-path jogging or walking. We also recommend changing the pace with Balance Walking, increasing the pace or a light jog for interval training. This will kick your Balance Walking program to even higher levels.

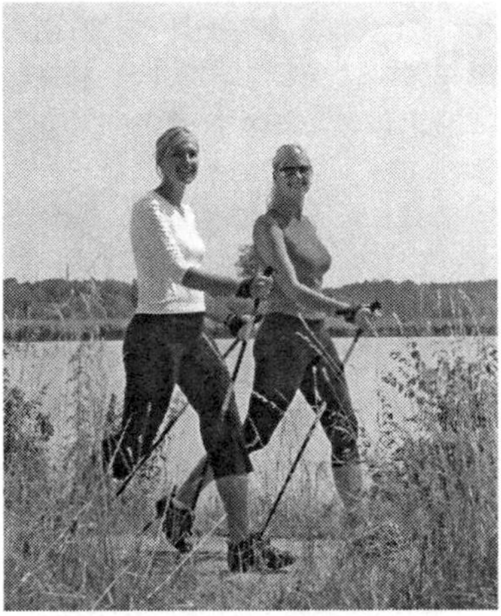

**Q:** I want to lose cellulite. Will Chung Shi and Balance Walking help me to do that?

**A:** There is a lot of debate about whether one can actually lose cellulite or not. For those who believe one can, the principle belief is that increased circulation decreases cellulite. Balance Walking increases circulation. The Chung Shi Balance Step is actually classified by the European Union (EU) as a medical device for the specific purpose of improving circulation. Chung Shi specifically works the muscles of the legs and buttocks, firming up the areas where cellulite tends to occur. There is no question that you can change the appearance of cellulite and you will notice the difference. We have had a number of Balance Walkers say it has worked for them.

**Q:** Why use Chung Shi shoes for Balance Walking?

**A:** Chung Shi shoes increase the workout level of Balance Walking. The increased range of motion achieved through Chung Shi increases your caloric burn rate, circulation as well as toning of legs, buttocks and abs. Couple this with well-documented Nordic Pole Walking benefits and you have a one-two punch to move your program to a level that is right for you and much more aggressive than regular walking.

**Q:** I have back and/or joint pain. Will Balance Walking help?

**A:** Yes. Balance Walking can be very helpful to those who suffer joint and back pain. The Chung Shi shoes put your body in an upright, aligned posture throughout standing, walking and jogging. The poles help to stabilize you and relieve pressure. In Chung Shi shoes, as on a natural surface, you keep your center of gravity over your ankles, pushing the ground behind you. 'Paved world gait', a Balance Walking technique, requires you to kick your leg out in front of you, heel strike, then, pull the ground towards you. This pulling gait causes the body to become stooped, creating misalignment and excessive strain at every step.

In Chung Shi shoes, you maintain an upright posture throughout the walking and running gait cycle. This means the vertebrae in your back stay on top of each other and the tendons, ligaments and muscles that support your joints are in alignment. So, the body is in a position to absorb the shock of standing and walking on the hard, flat surfaces of modern life more efficiently. And, with regular use of Chung Shi shoes, the muscles of the feet, legs, buttocks, abs and back are built up more evenly. In so doing, the more equally developed muscle structure then supports the upright, aligned posture, so that even when not wearing Chung Shi shoes, you'll stand up straighter and sit up taller!

And, the best part of Chung Shi shoes – you don't have to think about how to do it to get the benefit. Chung Shi shoes force the body into the aligned posture when standing, walking and jogging. So, just by putting on

Chung Shi shoes, you automatically gain relief for the back and joints.

**Q:** I have heel pain/forefoot pain. Will Chung Shi help?

**A:** Due to the unique, patented construction of the angled sole and rolling ramp, Chung Shi shoes redistribute pressure, requiring the mid foot to bear more weight, thereby reducing pressure at the heel and ball of the foot. When walking or jogging in Chung Shi shoes, the jarring forces at heel strike and toe-off are significantly reduced, therefore noticeably reducing or eliminating heel and forefoot pain. And, because of the gentle rolling motion of the shoe, Chung Shi shoes stretch the calf muscles and Achilles tendon, significantly helping those with a history of Achilles tendonitis, plantar fasciitis and heel spurs. This will allow you to continue your Balance Walking Program more comfortably.

**Q:** I have plantar fasciitis. Will this shoe help?

**A:** Chung Shi is an extremely effective tool for those suffering from plantar fasciitis. Because the plantar fascia (a tendon-like tissue) connects to the calcaneus (heel bone) at the very point where the foot strikes the ground with the most force at every step, simply walking in normal shoes can exacerbate the problem.

Chung Shi's unique sole significantly reduces force at heel strike, taking the pound out of every step. An ergonomically shaped stainless steel plate in the Chung Shi sole adds stability to the shoe, further supporting the plantar fascia. Additionally, because Chung Shi stretches the calf muscles, it loosens the Achilles tendon, which can also contribute to plantar fasciitis if not adequately stretched.

If there is pronation (the foot rolls inward) or supination (the foot rolls outward), an arch support may also be necessary to stabilize the foot medially/laterally (side-to-side) while using Chung Shi shoes. The experts at Foot Solutions can assist you with choosing the most effective arch support, if necessary. The objective is to keep you active and in the Balance Walking Program.

**Q:** I have diabetes. Will Chung Shi shoes help?

**A:** Chung Shi is very helpful to people with diabetes. It increases circulation and off-loads heel and forefoot pressure where problems often occur. It is often an important addition to diabetic foot health, provided that there is no history of ulcers or amputation on the feet. In cases such as this, it is important to consult with your medical professional prior to using Chung Shi. Furthermore, obtaining a physician's prescription will be required prior to dispensing Chung Shi shoes. If you are diabetic, the Balance Walking Program can have not only a significant impact on you, but a life-changing one. You will tone your body, reduce body fat and it will help you with your body chemistry. As a diabetic no matter what you do, please examine your feet daily especially if you are exercising. Remember, most diabetics have reduced flow of blood in their feet and can lose feeling. This is why you need to visually check your feet and identify the first signs of any issues. People with diabetes are at a very high risk for amputation but most can be prevented. Do your part!

**Q:** I am pregnant. Will Balance Walking help me to stay in shape and keep my feet and back feeling better throughout my pregnancy?

**A:** Yes. In addition to helping you keep in shape, Balance Walking puts the body in better alignment. This aligned posture takes pressure away from your back, hips, knees and feet, making those extra pounds more bearable. Chung Shi Comfort Step (Level One) is ideal for pregnant women.

However, because pregnant women should not start a new exercise program without consulting their physicians, we must ask that you provide a prescription from your doctor should you wish to purchase Chung Shi Balance Step (Level Two) shoes.

Also, please note that in your third trimester, your foot size will increase and it is very important for you to have shoes that will fit and support your feet properly. This will help gravity with lower back pain.

**Q:** Are there any activities for which I shouldn't wear Chung Shi shoes?

**A:** Yes. Chung Shi shoes are made for forward motion such as walking or jogging. Any sideways movement, such as tennis or aerobics, should be done in a sport-specific shoe, not Chung Shi. Further, when lifting heavy objects while standing (heavy free weights, moving the furniture in your house, etc.), you want a flat, stable base to control the lift. Chung Shi shoes are not flat, which is what makes the shoes work. But, that is also why you should not wear Chung Shi while lifting heavy objects.

For those of you who want to add the additional impact of balance to your workout, then Chung Shi shoes are the perfect workout partners. Or, if you are working out with light weights, you can use your Chung Shi shoes like a balance board.

**Q:** How long do they last?

**A:** Chung Shi shoes should last two to three times longer than your regular athletic shoes. Most shoes wear out at the heel and ball. Chung Shi bears most of the weight in the mid-foot, at the thickest point of the sole. Additionally, the soles of Chung Shi are made of polyurethane, which is a tougher material than the EVA that is typically used in traditional athletic shoes.

**Q:** Can I wear my arch supports with Chung Shi shoes?

**A:** Absolutely! And, you can even wear your arch supports in Chung Shi sandals, as they have a removable liner that will accommodate many shoe inserts. Arch supports are recommended for everyone that wants to improve their balance, performance, body alignment and stay active their whole life.

**Q:** How do Chung Shi shoes compare to other negative heel shoes?

**A:** Nothing compares to Chung Shi shoes. While some shoes have a negative heel and a mild rocker sole, they do not have the lever-like rolling ramp in the middle and the angled sole at the forefoot that is unique to Chung Shi shoes.

Chung Shi shoes are specifically designed to move the foot off the heel, through the mid foot and OFF THE TOE. Through Chung Shi's technology, you can achieve better alignment of the body and increased muscle use. The proper alignment that Chung Shi promotes is what creates the myriad of benefits of their use, from improving posture and building core stability to toning and strengthening muscles and alleviating joint and back pain.

**Q:** What should I focus on after I get them home?

**A:** Just begin slowly, gradually working up to wearing them full-time. You are changing the alignment of the body when wearing Chung Shi shoes. Therefore, you are shifting which muscles are working and how hard. To be conservative, it is suggested that you wear Chung Shi for an hour the first day. When you wake up the next day, listen to your body. If nothing is tired or sore, add an hour each day until you can comfortably wear Chung Shi shoes all the time.

If you wake up and are mildly sore, just don't increase the time that day, to give your body a chance to adjust to the workout. If you wake up and are notably sore, decrease the amount of time and add smaller amounts of time each day.

Additionally, you may choose to wear Chung Shi Comfort Step (Level One) for daily life to achieve the health and wellness benefits and wear Chung Shi Balance Step (Level Two) to maximize their daily Balance Walking routines.

**Q:** Why do they cost more than regular walking shoes?

**A:** The construction of the shoes is complex. They have an ergonomically shaped stainless steel plate, a fifteen or twenty degree sole (depending on which model) featuring a rolling ramp and use patented, state-of-the-art technology. Additionally, because of the way they are designed, Chung Shi shoes will last two to three times longer than traditional athletic shoes. As a result, you won't have to replace them as often as traditional athletic shoes.

Actually, for the many benefits of Chung Shi shoes and the fact that they will improve your posture as well as the way you look and feel, they are a bargain. It's time to put balance in your life!

After extensive testing I chose Chung Shi shoes for the Balance Walking program. Combine the many benefits of Chung Shi shoes with the many benefits of Balance Walking and you enter a new level of walking with not only increased benefits, but noticeable differences in toning and tightening of your legs, buttocks and arms. Add the improved posture and you will feel and look years younger in no time at all. Remember, this is about lifestyle changes that you can live with and will help you live a fuller and more active life.

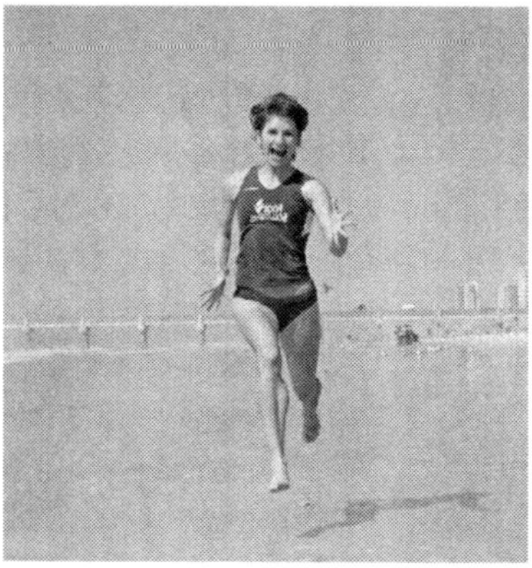

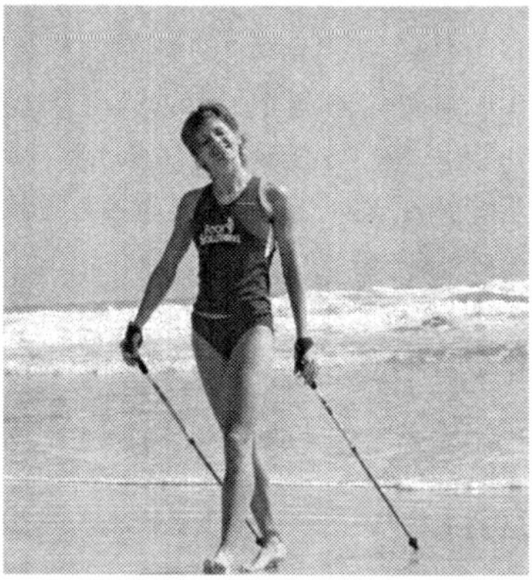

# Walking - Everyone Can Do It

Over seventy million people in the USA walk for exercise. Walking is a no-brainer and anyone can do it. The Asian philosophy on health is, "10,000 steps a day lead to a healthy mind and body." So, why don't we get off our butts and just do it? The biggest reason most people do not walk on a regular basis is that it is to time consuming and boring. Let's be realistic. There may be seventy million people walking, but we have all seen people walking and most of them do not depict a picture of good health or even walk at a pace that will accomplish any significant improvement. Let's face it! Time is our most precious commodity and we only have a limited amount, yet very few of us use it wisely. It stops for no one and we never have enough of it. Actually, this is really not true. Go back in time when you were a young child and you played outside from early morning until it was dark. The days were endless and it seemed like forever before you would be ten, then sixteen, then twenty-one, etc. Why were we all in such a hurry to be older to really enjoy life? Are you still on the same path now, waiting until you retire to do things you really should be doing now? Retirement is fine but remember, it is about the journey, so enjoy your whole life and do things in the moment.

This is not a problem that today's children have. Just look around you. There is everything from martial arts to swimming, dancing, music, and so on. Our children today are bored, inactive kids and yet, parents try to fill up their days with all sorts of outside activities. Look at the schedules many parents operate under, no wonder they are frazzled. What about the children? They are non-stop, morning-to-night, and most play time is computer games and TV. The most physically fit part of their bodies are their fingers from games and texting.

The simple point I am trying to make is that we are putting ourselves and our children into an endless cycle of racing through life. So, what is the answer? Slow down? Take long walks? We already know that this does not work.

So how about taking a hard look at life? Consider Balance Walking as a way to change your life... A low impact system that fifteen minutes a day can have significant impact on how you will feel and look.

Remember the Asian philosophy of 10,000 steps a day for healthy mind and body. With Balance Walking you can reduce this down to 5,000 steps. That is a 50% savings in time!

### Balance Walking

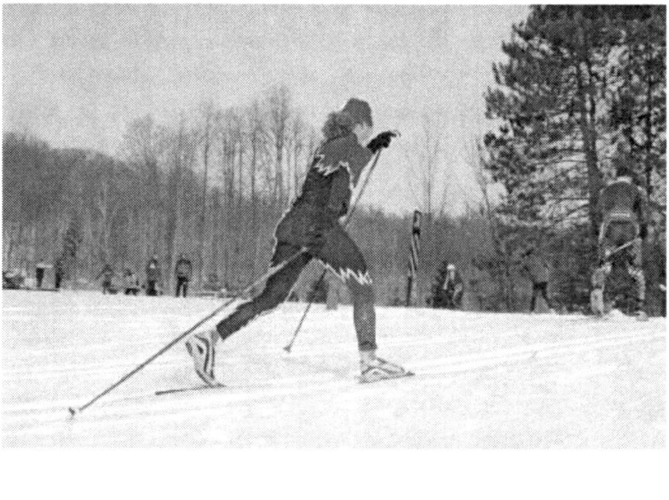

Pole walking has been around for years, a crossing over from cross-country skiing. It has been referred to by many names such as Nordic Walking, Pole Walking, and Ski Walking just to name a few. The most common referral is Nordic Pole Walking because of the popularity of cross-country skiing in this part of the world.

The roots of Nordic Pole Walking can be traced as far back as the 1930s as a summer cross-training method for top cross-country skiing athletes.

"Pole Walking" was introduced into a number of countries, to the public as an independent fitness activity that is extremely effective with many benefits over regular walking. In the '90s, Nordic Pole Walking experienced a boom in Finland and crossed over into mainstream exercise programs with an estimated 16% of the population participating. From Finland, it moved through Germany and Austria, and even to the land down under, Australia where they call it "Pole About." Nordic Pole Walking has just recently started to take hold in the United States.

## Health and Training Effects of Pole Walking

If you want to change your life and are interested in improving your health and appearance, you must exercise and make the commitment to a lifestyle change. The term, "use it or lose it," says it all. Your body is a complex biomechanical wonder; therefore it is of great importance to exercise on a regular basis, but in moderation. But most importantly, exercise should be fun! Cross-country skiing is one of the best sports for achieving a total-body workout, but can be too aggressive for most people. And it's especially difficult without snow. The proven advantages of cross-country skiing on the entire body and health are plentiful. For example, the stamina is improved, the majority of lower body muscles and all the upper body muscles (abs, chest, arms, back) are strengthened, and the immune system becomes more resistant. The trick is to get similar benefits without actually cross-country skiing.

Nordic Pole Walking is very similar to cross-country skiing in a number of ways, such as the movements, the health and training effects and benefits, and it can actually be done at any pace with results all year long, with or without snow in the forecast.

## Nordic Pole Walking – A Low-ImpactActivity For Everyone

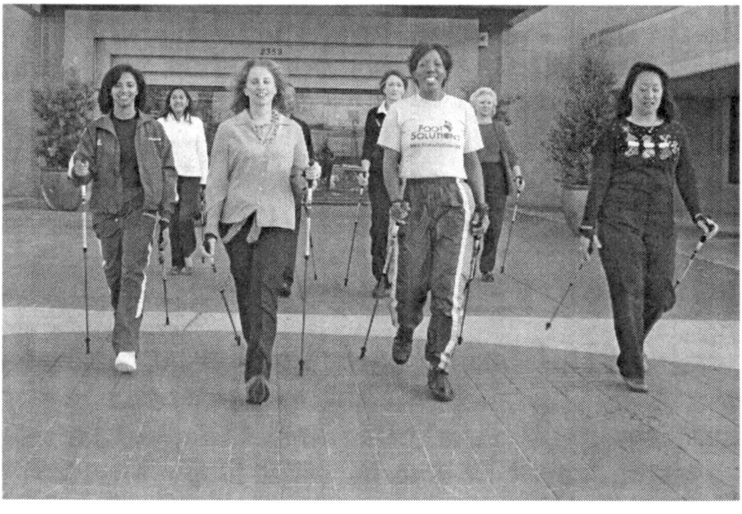

- Nordic Pole Walking activates and exercises 90% of all the human muscles through arm and upper body movement.

- Nordic Pole Walking is up to 46% more effective than walking without poles according to the study of Cooper Institute in Dallas.
- Nordic Pole Walking increases the burning of calories in comparison to walking without poles. The more work a person applies on the muscles, the higher the intensity is of the sport and the energy consumption of the human.
- Comparing jogging to Nordic Pole Walking, a large portion of strain can be transferred onto the poles, making this kind of sport very easy on the knees and ankles. For this same reason, Nordic Pole Walking is especially suitable for people with obesity and orthopedic problems like knee, hip or back pain.
- Nordic Pole Walking improves the blood circulation to the heart.
- Nordic Pole Walking does not only exercise the legs like walking or jogging, but provides the entire body a workout as well.
- Nordic Pole Walking increases the aerobic stamina while simultaneously strengthening the upper body muscles.
- Nordic Pole Walking reduces muscle strains and sprains in the shoulder and neck areas and prevents back pain. Especially people who are hunched over a desk benefit from this type of sport or exercise because it helps realign the body.
- Nordic Pole Walking is the optimal outdoor exercise for weight loss.
- Nordic Pole Walking increases the oxygen supply for the entire body through the active use of all the muscles used for breathing.

- Nordic Pole Walking is less tiring than jogging and reduces impact and jarring to the body, yet is not any less effective on the circulatory system.
- Nordic Walking improves your stamina and level of fitness.

## The Advantages of Nordic Pole Walking

- Nordic Pole Walking can be learned very easily and fast because it is a natural form of movement.
- Nordic Pole Walking provides a secure feeling while walking on uneven ground and represents a more secure walking option for elderly people.
- Nordic Pole Walking can be performed throughout the year anywhere.
- Nordic Pole Walking can also be performed in your neighborhood, at the park, the mall, etc. The poles are collapsible and travel very easily.
- The increased fat burning, strengthening and the toning of the upper body muscles make Nordic Pole Walking especially attractive to women.
- The small expenditure for material and supplies makes Nordic Pole Walking accessible to anybody.
- Nordic Pole Walking can be performed in any weather with the use of appropriate clothing.
- Nordic Pole Walking is normally found to be less tiring than classic-style walking and is a lot more fun to do.

- Nordic Pole Walking poles allow specific stretching and strengthening exercises to be performed, which would not be possible or effective enough without the poles. Having an exercise partner makes it possible to perform even more advanced exercises.
- The stretching and strengthening exercises with the poles, more specifically jumping and stepping routines, make the training interesting and versatile for beginning and advanced students alike.
- Nordic Pole Walking is a very controllable body activity. The intensity can be increased or decreased through the following methods:

  - Interval walking (fast/slow)
  - Use of hilly terrain
  - Step and jump exercises (walking, jogging, jumping, etc.)
  - The intensity of pressure used on the poles
  - Strengthening exercises

This makes Nordic Pole Walking interesting enough for beginners as well as professional athletes as an addition to their routine fitness program or a good foundation for their base program.

Nordic Pole Walking is ideal for new beginners and people who are starting back again, and those who are looking for an activity that is less demanding than jogging but more intense and fun than walking.

Nordic Pole Walking is now the fastest growing way to exercise across Europe for the masses. Germany has had an explosion in this area over the last 5 years. Now add the Foot Solutions Chung Shi shoes; scientifically designed with state-of-the-art technology. The combination of these techniques and technology now give you a program you can accomplish in minutes a day instead of hours, with increased benefits including burning more calories and increased muscle toning and shaping, especially in the leg and buttock areas.

Daily exercise is an important component for good health. Balance Walking using the Chung Shi shoe and the Nordic Pole Walking concept provides you with an option that will reduce your exercise time while, at the same time, increase benefits. This is an exercise program that is inexpensive and can be done all year long, with a group, alone or with your family. It is a fun way to add fitness to you and your family's daily lives. Do you like to walk with other people? Visit www.balancewalking.com to find a group near you!

# Too Good to be True

There are hundreds of studies and articles substantiating the benefits of Pole Walking. This includes articles by insurance companies in Germany that have used the program successfully to reduce medical claims and problems. Chung Shi shoes also have a number of supporting articles and testimonials on the benefits of the Chung Shi roller bar shoe. To find more information on studies visit our web sites, www.footsolutions.com or www.balancewalking.com You may also search the internet for Nordic Pole Walking and Chung Shi, to find a tremendous amount of research and validation of each component of The Balance Walking Way. It is the combination of each component that will give you a life changing transformation with a very small investment of time. It is important to address all four components to maximize your results.

Testimony from Dr. William Faddock, D.P.M.,CPED

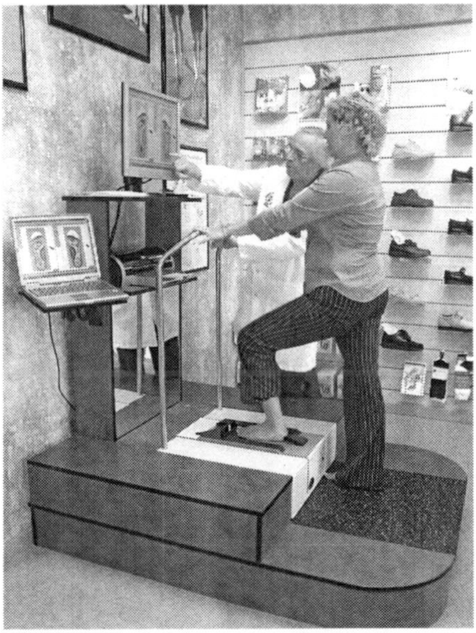

"Chung Shi is footwear we have long needed. I have treated patients with a wide array of foot and gait disorders. I have never seen footwear designed so perfectly to direct the feet and body through the correct biomechanical gait as Chung Shi. Chung Shi really will change the quality of life for so many who either wish to prevent problems or those in need of relief from painful conditions such as plantar fasciitis, metatarsalgia, Achilles tendonitis, various joint fusions, as well as the knee, hip and back disorders that trouble millions of us."

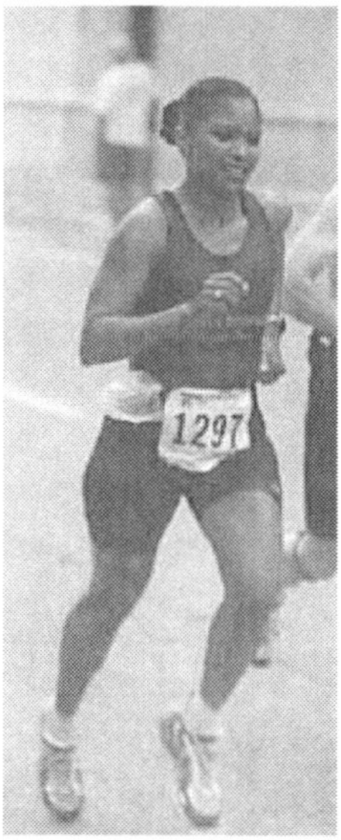


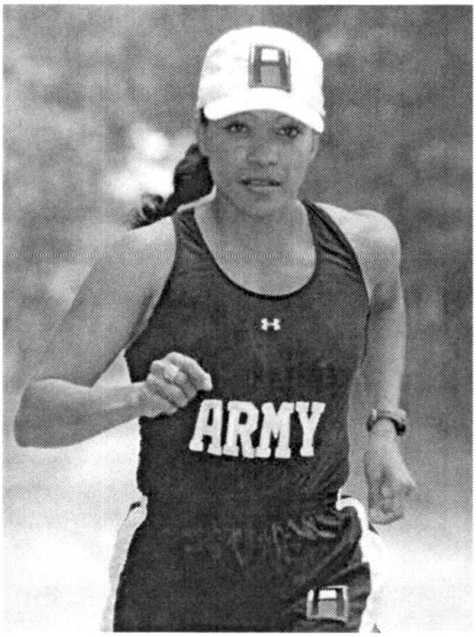


Foot Solutions' head running coach and Certified Nordic Pole Walking Instructor, Margaret Sue Bozgoz, is a retired U.S. Army Lieutenant Colonel, an all-Army marathoner, track runner and road racer who has coached ten's of thousands of walkers and runners. She has completed fifty-one marathons and too many road races to count. She started Nordic Pole Walking and coaching after retiring from the Army in the summer of 2006. Coach Bozgoz has been instrumental in testing and working with me on the Balance Walking program as well as successfully using Balance Walking as a recovery exercise after completing a marathon or triathlon for the Foot Solutions elite running team.

Studies show that training with Nordic poles increases cardiovascular activity and significantly enhances muscular and aerobic fitness. The sport was officially launched in 1997 but originated in the early 1930s in Finland when cross-country skiers started pole walking as a means to stay fit during their summer training.

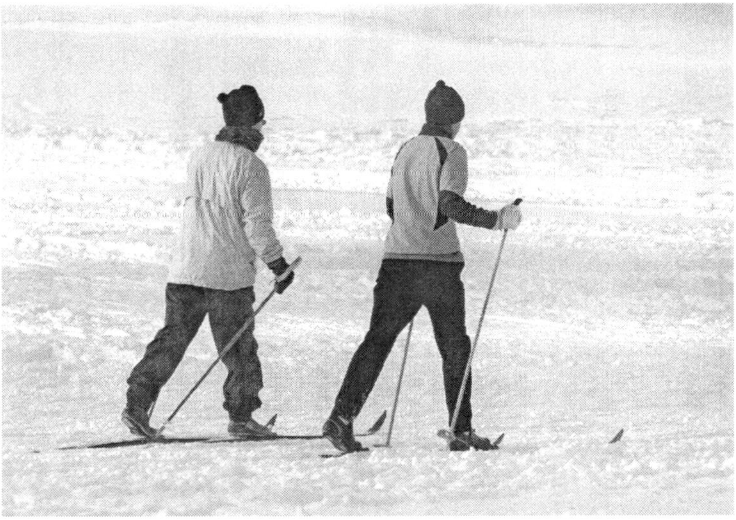

Today, approximately 760,000 Finns regularly participate in the sport. In addition, the trend has spread throughout Europe, where an estimated four million (4,000,000) plus people now participate in this sport on a regular basis. In North America, the sport is still relatively new, especially in the Southeast region.

In fact, Foot Solutions promotes free introductory classes for Balance Walking at all locations throughout the US and have hundreds of trained coaches to help get you started in this life changing experience.

"Balance Walking" combines all the benefits of Nordic Pole Walking with the advanced technology of Chung Shi shoes to actually increase the calorie burn process up to approximately 50% over regular walking, while improving body alignment and toning the legs, thighs and buttocks. What's more, it also gives you many more unbelievable health benefits and can be accomplished in just minutes a day!

## Getting Started

Before we get started on the Balance Walking technique, let's discuss the basic equipment you will need for your workout. It all starts with the poles. You cannot just use any poles; you will need a set that is specifically designed for pole walking. Our recommendation to start this program would be to use the Foot Solutions adjustable Balance Walking Poles. As the name suggests, they are adjustable, have a handy shoulder carrying case and best of all, they are relatively affordable. They will work well to get you started into the program without breaking the bank. In addition, Foot Solutions stores have a free introductory starter class with certified Nordic Pole Walking instructors. Visit www.footsolutions.com for more information on their walking program and the locations of their scheduled walks. If you want to try this out before investing in any equipment Foot Solutions and Balance Walking coaches provide loaner poles for your free lesson and walk.

You can also purchase your Chung Shi shoes and other Balance Walking needs at a Foot Solutions store or online, if there is not a convenient location in your area.

Working with a certified trainer will remarkably improve your walking technique and performance. However, if you are not located near a Foot Solutions store or one of the hundreds of trained coaches, we have a DVD available as well as an online video, showcasing the basic techniques of Nordic Pole Walking. Once you purchase your poles and Chung Shi shoes, you are ready to rock and roll!

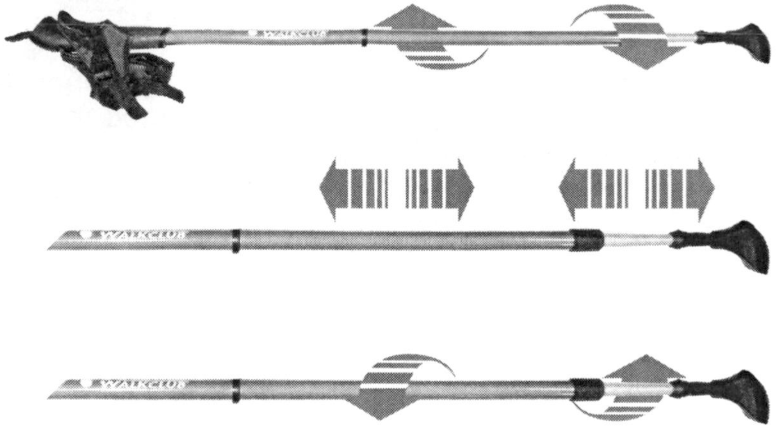

To start, you will need to adjust the length of the poles for your body height. While holding the pole by the handle, stand it upright on the floor in front of you. With your upper arm near your side and elbow bent to a 90° angle, tighten the pole adjuster so that the handle is even with your hand and the pole is parallel with your body. If you are a beginner we recommend you lower the pole another one to two inches so that the pole length is just under the ninety-degree 90° mark. This is a great way to help get your arms accustomed to the poles. As you get the rhythm and hang of it you can adjust the poles to the 90° mark. Please note: If you are doing off-road walking you should lengthen poles slightly, based on the terrain and ground type, and remove the rubber tip booty. When putting the booty back on, it should always point to the rear.

Once the poles have been adjusted, insert your thumbs into the hole of each wrist strap, paying attention to which is right and left, velcro them firmly, but comfortably around the wrist.

## Warming up

Balance Walking should always start with a warm-up to prepare your body for the walk and to help prevent injuries. The warm-up increases blood and oxygen circulation. In turn, this increases the flexibility of muscles and prepares you mentally and physically for your exercise session.

The walking poles are an excellent aid to increase your flexibility, strength and balance. Warm-up should start with a few minutes of walking and some warm-up exercises with your arms and shoulders. It is recommended that stretching should not be done at the beginning of your exercise program, but saved for the end when muscles have been warmed up and have better elasticity.

Keeping your body upright making sure not to lean forward and relax your shoulders and arms. Then, loosen your grip on the poles and hang you hands down to you sides. Casually start walking without gripping your poles. At this point, you are dragging your poles behind you. Walk about ten to twenty yards so you can just get the feel of walking while dragging the poles.

Next, grasp your poles loosely in order to gain control of them then gently swing your arms while you walk.

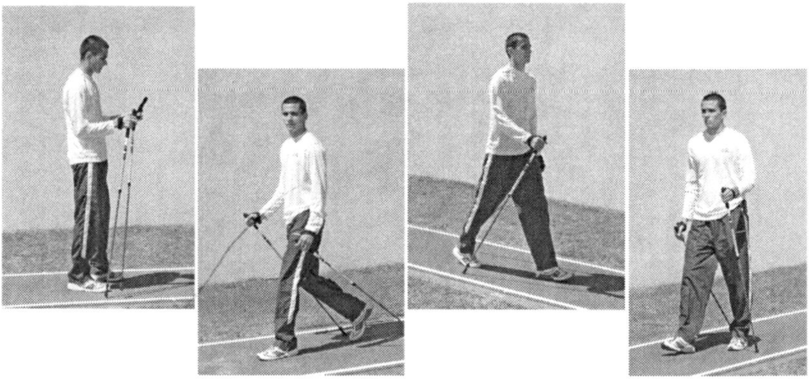

NOTE: The pole tips should not extend past the front of your feet as you walk. You are not reaching out; you are just swinging your arms. Do this for several minutes until you feel comfortable with the motion. If at anytime you feel out of rhythm, go back to dragging the poles for several steps. Remember that your shoulders must be down and relaxed so you are still walking in the correct posture and not leaning forward.

As you move the pole forward, plant and push off. At this point, the pole should be just above the ground and planted approximately one foot behind your lead foot. Your arms should not be fully extended, but slightly bent at the elbows. Walk like this until you feel very comfortable with your rhythm and stride.

The next step takes a little practice to get used to, but is a very important step to master. Remember, the pole is held with a comfortable grip but, and this is important, your grip should start to tighten just before you move the pole forward and plant it through the push-off. You then release grip as the pole moves behind you. This takes a little getting used to for most people. The more you think about it, the more you struggle with this phase. Just keep walking and let the grip-and-release technique come naturally.

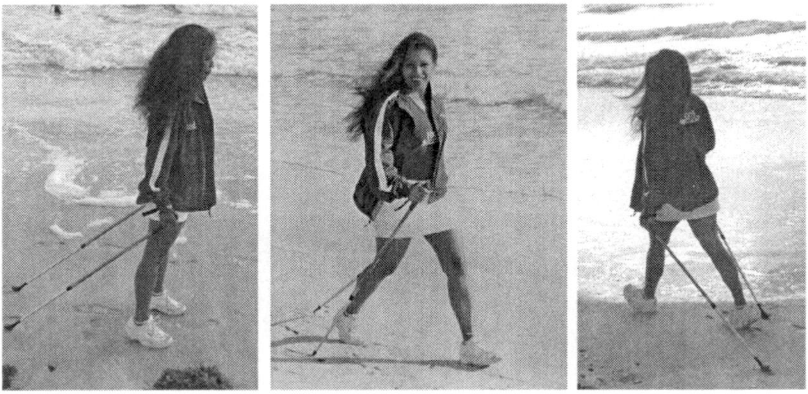

Mastering the grip-and-release technique is an important part of the process in order for you to achieve the full effect from your Balance Walking workout.

Once you are comfortable with your rhythm, you can concentrate more on swinging your arms and actually get your shoulders into the arm-swinging movement. Again, your body and shoulders should be in a relaxed, correct posture position. Congratulations! You have just mastered the basic Nordic Pole Walking technique!

Remember, Balance Walking is a low-impact fitness walking system used to create a total body workout without taking a toll on your body. You will be working the large muscle groups of both your upper and lower body. Along with toning your arms, shoulders, chest, buttocks and leg muscles, you will also be getting a heart pumping cardiovascular workout. Balance Walking will improve your whole body as well as the state of your mind.

Balance Walking can be done anywhere and during any season, which is what is so great about this form of exercise.

If weather is a problem, the mall is a great place to walk. Most malls have walking times from 7am to 10am, before the stores open.

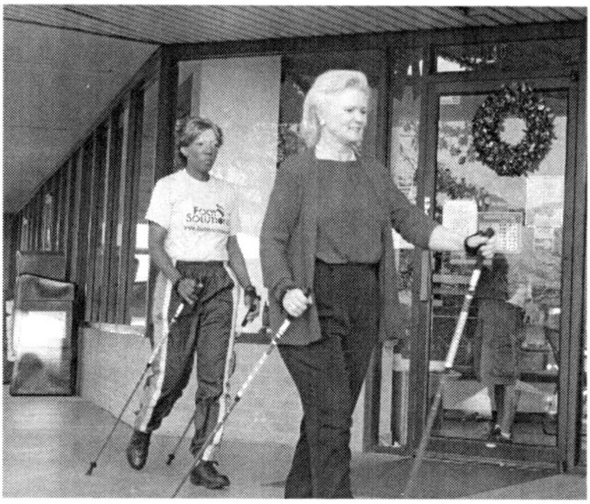

You will notice the rubber tips located on the end of your walking poles. These are removable for off-road walking in rough terrain or on the trail. The rubber tips are also easily replaced, should they become worn or damaged.

Listed below are some common beginner's mistakes to watch out for:

- 'Death grips' on the poles will create tension up your arms and neck. Looking down at your feet will affect your posture. Have your chin up, shoulders back and relaxed.
- Putting the poles in front of your feet and body – You should always push behind you with the poles, instead of reaching and extending your arms like pistons in an engine – push, push, push.
- Wrongly using the same leg with the same pole, making your stride feel weird and off. Just as with regular walking, each hand should meet its opposite foot to keep your stride in balance.
- Thinking too hard about the movement - Your body will know how to do it because it is natural.

Balance Walking itself is not difficult. You already have fifty percent of it down if you know how to walk! However, there are some things to which you must pay attention. You will want to maintain correct upright posture; be sure not to reach out with the poles and do not over-extend your step. This is more about finesse and proper technique.

Remember, when you get off the beat, just stop moving the poles and drag the poles again for several minutes until you get your rhythm back. There is no rush and no competition. Just keep going back to basics whenever needed. Even experienced pole walkers have to stop and drag their poles to get the rhythm back. Once you've got it, it's intuitive, fun and a fabulous workout.

Now, let's get into some additional techniques that you will find useful as you expand your program.

## BALANCE WALKING – FAST MODE

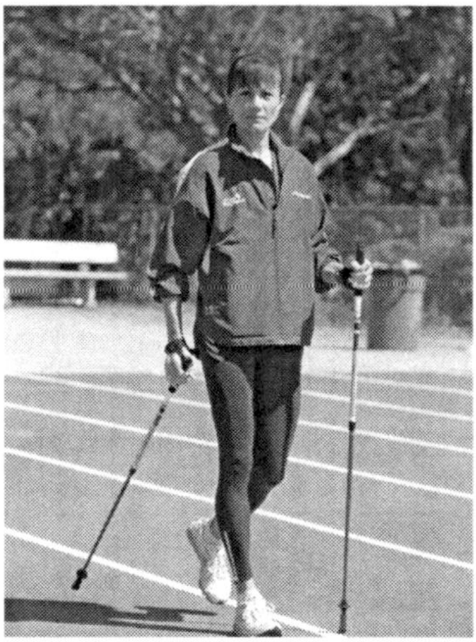

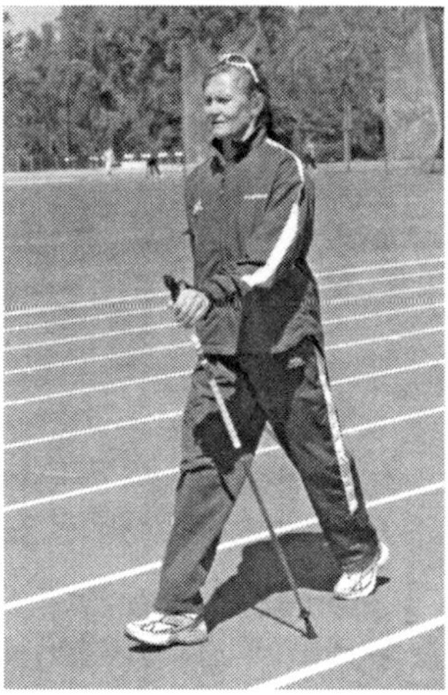

Speeding up your pace should not cause you to break form; you still want to maintain good posture and rhythm. You are not taking bigger steps; you are taking faster steps. This means that your body rhythm must keep up with your feet. This is natural and once you have mastered the basic Balance Walking technique, it should not be a problem. A great way to practice this is with short interval training.

Walk with a fast pace for two minutes then fall back to a regular pace for eight minutes. As your stamina increases, you can adjust your speed burst accordingly. Remember, this is not a race. It is all about you, how you feel and what you want to accomplish with your Balance Walking routine.

## BALANCE WALKING – JOGGING

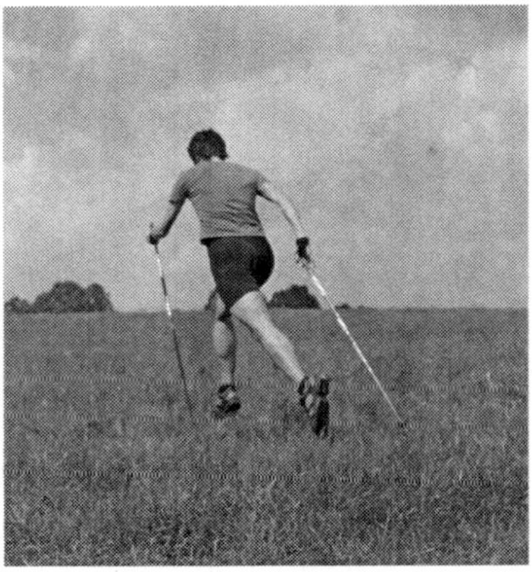

Yes, you can increase the tempo to a light jog, again using the poles for rhythm and control. You can occasionally throw in a light jog if you wish to increase your workout pace or level. This is not necessary or required. I only mention it for the aggressive exercisers who always want to push the envelope. The poles can be used effectively to take some of the strain off your knees and back which is one of the reasons injured runners like it.

## BALANCE WALKING – GLIDING

This occurs when you are gracefully gliding (think of a gazelle-like action) one foot to the other. In this case, you are almost running, but moving more smoothly with less of an impact on your joints. Again, this will get your heart rate up and is suggested only for the physically fit that want to take it to the highest level.

For the competitive junkie, fast mode, jogging and gliding will test your endurance and the rest of your body. For most of us, good-old, basic Nordic Pole Walking with some speed intervals will be enough.

When walking with other people, it is important for the group to break up into Balance Walking levels. Slower beginners in one group with advanced in another. This allows people to enjoy the walk at a level appropriate for their skill set and their individual goals. Walking groups and partners make the walks more entertaining; I have actually held business meetings and discussions during walks that have been very fruitful. Since I am an acknowledged workaholic I feel like I am taking care of two issues at the same time. Talk about efficiency!

## BALANCE WALKING – UP HILL

While going uphill, place the body in a position that is bent slightly forward and plant the pole alongside your lead foot. You will be using your arms and upper-body strength more while putting the added pressure on the poles. Your whole body will get a more aggressive workout. As a result, hills should be included in your workouts as you progress.

## BALANCE WALKING – DOWN HILL

What goes up must come down. Going downhill requires shorter steps. Also, the poles should be planted just in front of the foot and with the added pressure you're putting on the pole, less pressure will be placed on the legs and knees which is especially beneficial to those with bad or weak knees.

The basic Balance Walking techniques will allow you to safely walk at your own pace and on any terrain, whereas the more advanced techniques are designed to bring your workout to the next level. Remember, the primary principle of the poles is not only to increase your workout intensity by using 90% of your muscles, but will allow you to use the poles to take the pressure and weight off the rest of your body and help with core stability.

This balancing effect allows you to participate in a program even if you are overweight, have minor mobility problems or medical issues. You can be young or old, in great shape or just trying to find your way back to a healthy lifestyle.

Remember, this program is about you and your present activity level. Put balance back into your life with a Balance Walking program that is designed for your needs and level of activity.

## COOL DOWN

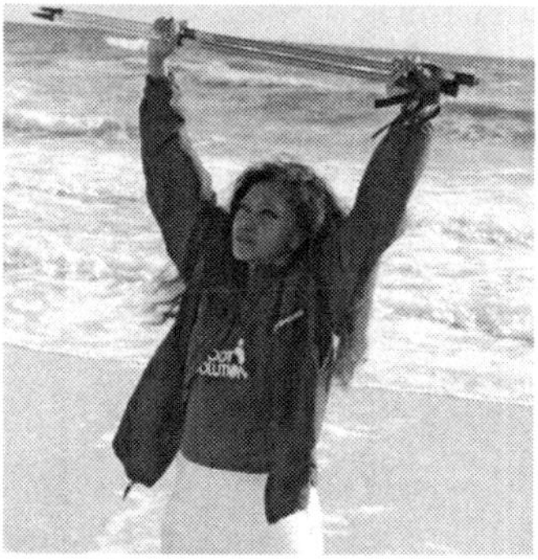

This is an important part of your program and can be as simple as winding down your walk for the last several minutes and finishing with some basic stretching techniques. Stretching is best performed when your body is thoroughly warmed up. Gentle stretching will help you stay flexible and more youthful.

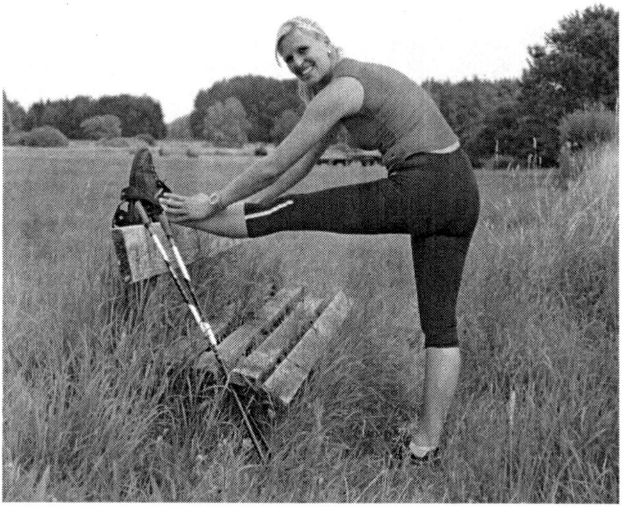

# What People are Saying about Nordic Pole Walking

## Nordic Walking Poles, a Fitness Trend for Walkers of All Ages, Sizes and Fitness Levels

Nordic Walking Poles are fast becoming a year-round, worldwide fitness trend. While the virtues of using poles are well known among those who hit the ski slopes, use of Nordic Walking Poles are making their way to walking and hiking trails, neighborhoods, beaches, tracks and even shopping malls.

The concept of Nordic Pole Walking originated many years ago in Finland as Olympians sought out year-round training options. Today, an estimated 100,000 Americans enjoy Nordic Pole Walking, and an estimated four million enjoy the sport across Europe.

Coach Sue Bozgoz, Foot Solutions Master Certified Nordic Pole Walking Coach has been trained by German Nordic Pole Expert Dr. Klaus Schwanbeck and president of Nordic Pole Walking USA and former Olympic trainer in Germany. I also had the opportunity to Nordic Pole walk with Klaus and to discuss at length the benefits of Nordic pole walking and his extensive training experience in Germany and here in the US.

Bozgoz uses pole walking as a recovery exercise after marathons or triathlons for all her runners and says pole walking is a great way to enhance all-over fitness.

"With proper use, Nordic Poles allow an individual to use 90% of their total body muscles," says Bozgoz. "The poles provide a great benefit whether walking for health or for someone looking for new ways to intensify an existing fitness program."

Nordic walking poles were designed from cross country ski poles to be used on a variety of surfaces without cross country skis. The poles are lighter and contain straps that enclose the palm of the hand, similar to fingerless gloves, and they have removable rubber tips. Walking with Nordic poles can burn up to 46% more calories than traditional walking, and use of the poles helps posture and body alignment. In addition, core muscles are strengthened, assisting total body conditioning as well as enhancing cardiovascular circulation.

Mike Dickie, a fifty-four year-old diabetic from Atlanta, Georgia, started using Nordic walking poles to help maintain his blood sugar levels and as a fitness routine after heart surgery. His sixteen year-old daughter, also a diabetic, joined in and both use a Nordic walking program to maintain a healthy lifestyle. Says Dickie, "In addition to helping keep my blood sugar levels more stable, we've both noticed benefits in our overall fitness level and posture. We've enjoyed the walking/talking time together. My wife, a school nurse, joins in on a regular basis."

Dr. Art Lee, a heart surgeon at Grady Hospital in Atlanta, Georgia, adds, "The Nordic poles provide a low impact and joint friendly mechanism for my patients. Post-surgery individuals, many of whom are older or obese, benefit from physical activity, and Nordic walking poles are a perfect tool to get these people moving safely and efficiently. It's also a stress and tension reducer, which is important to recovery."

According to Dr. Klaus Schwanbeck, President of Nordic Pole Walking USA, "Pole Walking is the most effective all-around low-impact exercise targeting the broadest population." Traditional walking is the single largest category in the sporting goods market in the U.S. with an estimated eighty-six million Americans participating. Adding Balance Walking to this market can improve fitness, health and wellness to millions of Americans.

Dr. Klaus Schwanbeck, the president of Nordic Pole Walking USA has been involved in the certification process for Nordic Pole Walking in Germany and now here in the USA. Foot Solutions has over 200 stores nationwide, hundreds of certified Balance Walking coaches and is represented in twelve countries, providing state-of-the-art technology to assess and evaluate foot issues and body alignment. Foot Solutions also offers free introductory Nordic Pole Walking classes and supports hundreds of scheduled walks across the country. Please visit www.footsolutions.com to see where the closest coaches and locations are to you. Also visit the online shopping site for products and DVDs if there is not a convenient location to you.

I have personally studied and reviewed Nordic Pole Walking with experts from Europe, Australia, Canada and the United States. All techniques are very similar and the validation of daily practitioners around the world make Nordic pole walking a proven concept. There are literally thousands of documents and testimonials for web surfers that may be interested in details and outside validation.

## Fitness Trend for the New Millennium

Balance Walking: the activity for anyone, anywhere, any age and any lifestyle. Balance Walking is inexpensive. Learn how now and walk with our well-established network of coaches and classes. Not close to one of our free introductory classes? Visit our website for online information on how to establish your own program and don't forget our DVDs and online activity tracking system to monitor your progress and results.

## Anyone can do this - Age is not a barrier.

The poles improve balance and stability, making you more confident, as you continue to strengthen and tone. Feel fit and fabulous while you walk. Balance Walking could be the fountain of youth we've all been searching for, a simple approach built on well-proven components that have been around and available for years. The answers and solutions have always been there. But most of us are too busy and constantly looking for the easy way out. We must accept responsibility and we must implement change in our life. This is a simple approach that does not take much time and could have a significant impact on each one of us.

Children love Balance Walking too. They can walk, run, jump and train simply and safely, making this sporting activity a family affair that can bridge the generation gap. We have introduced it to schools and camps. Children have short attention spans and regular walking just doesn't work for them. They get bored too quickly. I even get bored with regular walking!

Are you out of shape or inactive? No problem. This is truly a low-impact activity that is enjoyed by all fitness levels. From the couch potato to the elite athlete, Balance Walking will help you get into the next level and more importantly, keep you there. You may need more stability, more time or you may be in great shape and want to push the envelope.

# Balance Walking & Food

As we all know, there is so much data available on food diets and quick weight loss programs. However, most do not work over time. My heritage is Italian, and as I was growing up, food was an important part of the celebration of life. So, let's start by eliminating the word "diet" and stop thinking about it. How about using common sense instead?

Part of the problem is when you start playing games with food and try all the shortcut methods to lose weight; you actually throw off the natural balance of your body. The real secret to success in this area is not really a secret at all. It is simple: eat and enjoy life! Over time, your eating habits should evolve to adjust to your particular body needs. Food is one of the pleasures of life and punishing yourself is just not going to work.

What does work? It is quite simple. Consider a form of grazing. For example, try eating smaller meals four to five times per day. Another option would be to have three meals a day with small snacks in between and before bedtime to keep the fire burning. If weight is an issue for you, eat six times a day. You can double your fat loss with this technique.

## Breakfast the one meal you should NEVER miss!

It is well documented that eating breakfast will help you lose weight and actually keep you from gorging out later. Also, if you feel as though you need to eat a large meal everyday, be sure to make it lunch instead of at the end of the day, similar to what they do in the Mediterranean countries. Let us take a look at the single biggest issue in eating - portion control and the amount of chemicals and fillers in the food we eat.

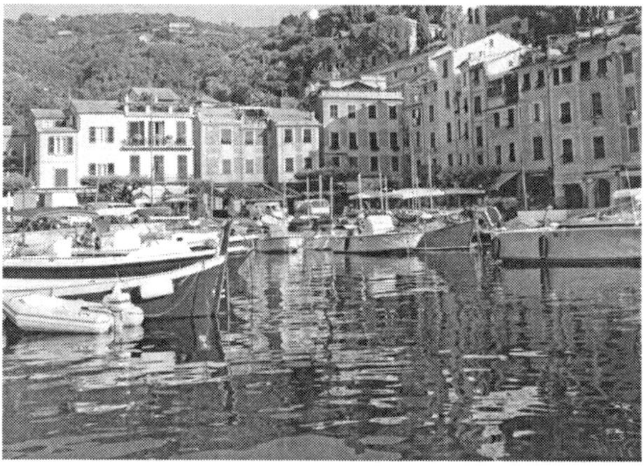

On a recent trip to Italy I had wonderful meals that were so tasty and fresh but the key was they were reasonable portions. I did not hesitate to eat anything and never felt stuffed like I normally do here in the US. In addition it has been well documented that drinking red wine is healthy. In fact the longest living Europeans drink red wine their whole lives and yes, I drank red wine at every meal and it felt great!

Sticking with an exercise and eating plan that you can live with, is what Balance Walking is all about. This is a lifelong decision and does not end when you reach your goal. Losing weight short-term is easy. It is keeping the weight off over time that becomes the issue.

Forget about low fat and substitute chemicals. Think natural and eat the real foods instead of trying to trick your body with substitutes that are not healthy for you and really don't accomplish anything. Just look around you at all the wonder diets, pills and low-fat products. If they are working, how come obesity is increasing instead of decreasing?

If you want to change your life and live a more, healthy, full lifestyle, then you have to be willing to make these simple commitments. Enjoying Balance Walking for as little as 15 minutes a day for three to four days a week, combined with following a reasonable, healthy eating program without starving yourself will give you remarkable results. Remember, we are talking about a lifestyle change. This is not a quick fix, but an investment in yourself for the way you will live the rest of your life.

An additional basic part of the problem is portion control. You must realize that you cannot eat huge portions without paying the price. There are many ways to overcome this problem. Learn to recognize a reasonable portion size. The size of your palm is equal to one portion size. Most meals are comprised of 3 portions which include 1 protein, 1 vegetable and 1 natural grain.

Also, use smaller plates instead of oversized ones like those used in restaurants that serve one-size meals. Unfortunately, in the United States, it is more about quantity than quality. Cut your portions in half and save the other half for another meal. Also, take your time while eating. Try tasting and chewing, your food, instead of wolfing it down. Give your body a chance to let you know it is no longer hungry. Drink water before and during your meal. Most Asian cultures have a cup of soup before their meals and drink hot tea with their meals. It works! Also, simple things like portioning your meal and putting the food away so you don't continue eating. Family-style eating with continuing oversized portions makes it easy to overeat. Family-style works if you use the Chinese approach; it's about the taste; you take a small serving from each plate. If you don't, there won't be anything left for the rest of the group. It is about experiencing the many wonderful tastes and textures. If you do have an opportunity to eat with a Chinese family, they always take small portions and insure the elders at the table get first choice. It is a great tradition and will earn you respect.

If weight is a problem for you, weigh yourself everyday, it is best to weigh yourself at the same time of each day for consistency, i.e. every morning. However, be sure you do not obsess over ounces. You are catching small changes as they occur so that your weight does not spiral out of control. Stop punishing yourself if you eat something you enjoy. Instead, learn to celebrate the moment and to enjoy each occasional indulgence. The more you make of it, the harder it will become to control and the urge will become a constant struggle. Trying to eliminate favorite foods is the wrong approach; you will always feel deprived. You are much better off eating it. Try eating sensible portions and really take your time, chewing the food thoroughly, enjoying the taste and the texture. Slow yourself down; life is simple. Try to learn good eating habits, but know that it is okay to indulge occasionally, provided that you make the most of the moment. When it comes to steering clear of certain items, make sure over-processed flour and sugar are at the top of your list. For some reason most of these products seem to settle at the waist. The eating issue is really very simple; you either, burn and process what you eat or it will stay with you until you do. The better level of fuel (food) that you put into your body will make it easier to burn and give you more energy. If you use improper fuel, your engine will react badly, just like in your car. Have you ever followed a car that is choking on itself and spitting out smoke? The same goes for your body.

Eating right does not take rocket science. It is about making some sensible changes and returning to a more natural way of living. It is about eating well and living well; think natural, healthy, quality, taste and smaller wonderful meals. The trick is to get away from processed convenience foods and the absurd quantities. Try cooking simple, but healthy meals; they really are a strong part of enjoying life. Try eating with friends and family and make it a time to communicate with each other. Take the time to talk between bites to slow everything down. You will develop stronger and better relations with your friends and family and may realize that this is really a great part of life.

Shift to essential building blocks. Simple meals mean fresh, natural ingredients. Use some organic ingredients and purchase local items in season.

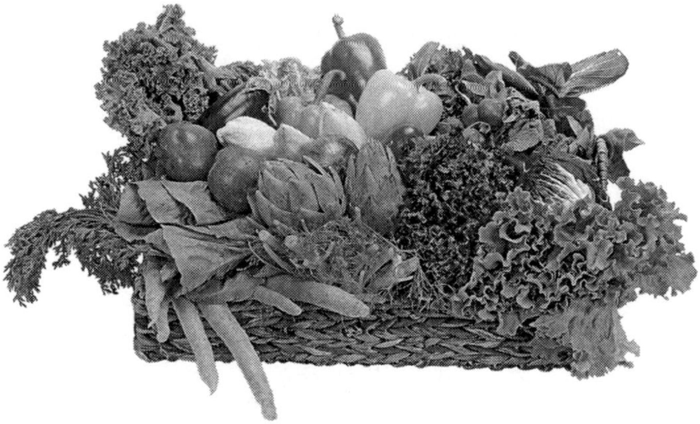

Check your pantry or fridge and get rid of high fat and highly processed foods, use more fruits and vegetables. Try mixing grains and beans together; they form a complete protein and have been a basic staple for centuries.

There is no restriction on what you eat provided you pay attention to the quantities, eating 4 to 5 smaller meals a day. When possible, try to include healthy and fresh foods in your daily diet.

Proteins – include lean meats, poultry, fish, eggs or protein powder.

Dairy – includes milk, cheese and yogurt.

Vegetables – includes any vegetable that is green or you would eat raw.

Starch – includes whole grains, wild rice and potatoes (sweet is healthier).

Fat – whether you realize it or not, yes, fat is essential and necessary for healthy and balanced eating. Be sure you do not eat the wrong ones. Stick with olive oil, butter, nuts and seeds.

Fruit – the list for this category is endless and can help satisfy many urges for something richer and more fulfilling. It is the natural way to satisfy those cravings for something sweet and the possibilities are endless.

**NOTE** – We are not talking about calorie counting or restrictions. Think spices, more exotic fulfilling dishes. Think European or Asian. If you have traveled outside the U.S., the first thing you probably noticed is the reasonable portions that were served and consumed by the locals. Food is about the senses, how it looks, how it smells, how it feels in your mouth and how good it tastes. Taste is not about speed; it is about enjoying the moment. One time in France, while eating a wonderful dessert, I was told by a local that I did not eat it, I swallowed it; they were right. They were enjoying the burst of flavors and wonderful feeling of this dessert while I inhaled it. Lesson learned: It is not the amount that is satisfying, but that burst of flavor; savor it and enjoy it.

Eat 4 to 5 meals a day and never skip breakfast. Make sure to include two servings from each group and if you want more, make it more vegetables and fruit. Rethink your plate; have 4-5 ounces of quality meat or fish, 4 ounces of legumes or whole grains and 4 ounces of vegetables. No seconds – enjoy this plate of food, eating more often takes the edge off and will help keep you from over indulging. For dessert have fruit; use your imagination. Did you know that it is estimated that less than 33% of the population are eating the recommended servings of fruit and vegetables a day? Select natural, nutritious food loaded with healthful amino acids, vitamins and minerals, try to eliminate overly processed foods and foods loaded with unnatural substitute products. The solution has always been right in front of us. We have just chosen convenience and quick fixes over what has worked successfully for generations before us. Food and meals used to be a chance to get together and enjoy the moment. The meal could be simple, but the ingredients were fresh and tasty. Actually, cooking should also be part of the process, then taking the time to enjoy the meal and the company. Today, most of us live and rush through life and eat what will fill the void the quickest. Families hardly ever eat together anymore; everyone has something more important to do.

Just look back at the statistics, twenty-five years ago; then fifty years ago:

When I was in school there was one kid in class that was overweight. Today when you visit a classroom, 1/3 are very overweight. Another 1/3 are borderline. Listen to the stories on TV; listen to the news and all the changes that are being suggested to correct childhood obesity. Worse yet, they try to blame it on someone else. The solution is simple; don't buy stuff that is bad for you and the problem will be solved. As a business person, if most of my customers want a hamburger or any other dish loaded with fat, that is what I would sell them. Don't blame me; order something else. And as a business person I will adjust my menu immediately to accommodate my customers in order to stay in business.

We must go back to basics and common sense. We must forget about the miracle solutions; they do not exist. There is so much information on foods and diets that most people have information overload. Focus must be placed on the four groups of food and how to enjoy them. Remember, a little fat is healthy and will help you lose weight as long as you stay away from the substitutes. Have you ever wondered what goes in all those products with zero fat and reduced calories?

If you want more information on food and meal planning, please visit our website at www.BalanceWalking.com.

Eating well is part of the Balance Walking Way lifestyle change, without it you may always struggle to achieve the results you need in order to live a happy, healthy, more active life. Besides, it has been determined through a number of studies that stress and lack of sleep will add significantly to your weight issue and many other health-related problems. For this reason, Balance Walking focuses on having balance in one's life.

## Water – Water – Water

### Water is Life

Water is necessary for life and if you want to achieve control of your weight flushing your system with water every day is a basic requirement for healthy living. Basic requirements is 8 to 10 glasses of water a day, if you are over weight you should add an additional glass for every 25lbs over weight you are.

Water is the body's most important nutrient, is involved in every bodily function, and makes up 70-75% of your total body weight.

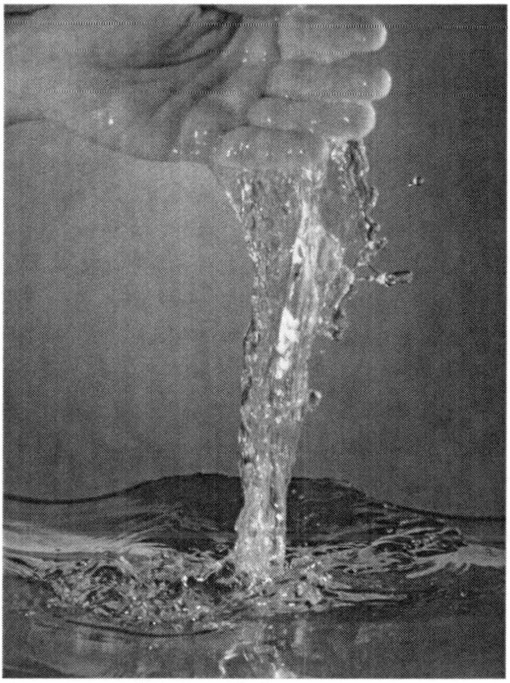

Coffee, soda, wine, these liquids do not count as water intake and will not purge your system.

Want an extra cleanser for your body? Add a teaspoon of apple cider vinegar to a few of these glasses or some fresh lemon juice.

Another way to help is to have a bowl of soup before your main meal or snack, something simple, chicken, vegetable, etc. Not cream or thickened soup, think simple and basic. Soup is a staple in the Far East there are good reasons to start the meal with some soup.

If you are not a water drinker now start off by adding a extra glass to your intake over a 10 day period, you should be able to reach a level of water intake to balance and flush your system. You will feel the difference and the majority of people do not drink enough water.

## Children & Obesity

On the July 3, 2000 issue of NEWSWEEK magazine, the cover featured children with a headline reading, "FAT FOR LIFE" and included an article about six million kids who are seriously overweight. What can we do?

Today, the fat epidemic for kids continues, with an estimated eight million children and adolescents who are overweight. These numbers are substantial and based on current trends. Thirty-three percent of children born in the year 2000 will develop Type II Diabetes.

Medical studies indicate that this could be the first generation where children will die before their parents. As a parent, these numbers are alarming, not to mention the additional medical costs and quality of life this generation will need to face.

There is no strategic national or state policy to combat obesity and physical inactivity. Obesity rates for both adults and children have more than doubled since 1980. "Lack of funding" is the excuse that is being used as the number one barrier to addressing the growing problem of obesity?

Both the medical community and the county officials are beginning to recognize that childhood obesity is a serious public health problem, an issue that increases morbidity and mortality, having substantial medical, economic and social costs.

How many articles and studies do people need to wake up? It is estimated that medical costs and lost worker productivity, as a result of obesity, is approximately 117 billion dollars and 27% of health care costs are directly associated with obesity. We live in a country of convenience and quick fixes. What makes it worse is that we are to blame for the position in which we have placed ourselves, and if we as parents and a nation wait for someone else to solve the problem, it is not going to happen. NOTE: OBESITY WILL NOT GO AWAY BY ITSELF AND WILL CONITNUE TO GET WORSE, NOT BETTER.

I find it humorous that everyone is looking for someone to blame. Some of the most common scapegoats include the government, workplace, community, schools, fast food, television, computer games, vending machines, cafeterias, food manufacturers, and the list goes on.

NEWS FLASH: The only person to blame is YOU! We will expand this to the primary culprits, your parents. This is where it starts, and ultimately there is really no one else you can blame.

Please stop blaming businesses and the government for your problem. Businesses exist to make money, if you buy it they will sell it. If you want healthier, better quality foods then establish the need, and believe me, the businesses will respond. The government is not the cause or the one to blame for our society's eating problems.

## So, what is the solution?

Actually, the solution is very simple and has always been available. Control portion size and eat smaller meals more often throughout the day. In addition, you must know that what you eat is important. The same healthy guidelines that have been displayed in the pyramid of recommended food choices for years are all you need. They include lean meat, fish and chicken, vegetables, grains, fruit and nuts. Don't forget a little fat is not only healthy, but also necessary. Think of your body as a sophisticated engine. Engines run on fuel so the food you eat drives that engine. If you don't drive your car for a while, if you don't take the care to put in the proper fuel, what happens? Yes, the engine becomes sluggish, it doesn't feel right, and it may not even start. Think of your body the same way. The major difference: you can replace your car, but you are stuck with your body for the rest of your life. Do you want a body that will carry you effortlessly through the rest of your life? Do you want to be active when you are older and enjoying your life to the fullest? I know these are really foolish questions. The problem is that most of us have been ignoring them.

DIETING AND QUICK FIXES REALLY DO NOT WORK. This has been proven over and over again. Why do you think every year there is a new wonder diet or pill that will solve all your problems? Even body creams that you rub on your body to make fat disappear! What is really amazing is all the television shows on losing weight and the ridiculous lengths people will subject themselves to in order to try and get results.

Think about lifestyle changes that you can live with. Eating is one of the most wonderful gifts of life; food should be enjoyed and considered a celebration of life. Return to family values and enjoying the company of family and friends with good food and conversation. Turn off the TV and make this a family time to talk with each other and find out what is happening in your family's lives. You need to establish lifestyle changes that are right for you. This should include some form of activity such as Balance Walking, which is simple, inexpensive, and can be done anywhere, any time, alone or with family, friends or exercise groups. You should also give yourself a small amount of quiet time each day to just let your mind help rejuvenate itself. Just five minutes a day of quiet time and another fifteen minutes of Balance Walking coupled with basic nutritional common sense is enough to change your life.

## Fitness

The physical fitness part of Balance Walking may be described as cross-country skiing without the skis, exercising the entire body and encouraging an upright posture and balance without placing unnecessary stress on the muscles, ligaments and tendons. Participants use modified ski poles and specially designed Chung Shi shoes.

The bottom line: Balance Walking allows walkers to use their entire body while maintaining perfect posture and burning approximately fifty percent more calories.

## Health benefits of Balance walking

- Provides education on preventing health issues and increases total body workouts
- Develops upright posture and proper body alignment
- Burns up to 50% more calories than conventional walking
- Enhances cardiovascular performance
- Improves overall body alignment
- Improves strength and endurance
- Simultaneously provides an upper-body workout
- Improves balance and stability

- Minimizes stress and force to feet, shins, knees, hips and back
- Helps develop a positive body image, self-esteem and self confidence
- Develops overall physical/psychological development
- Fosters social development
- Offers a positive pastime and healthy source of amusement for participants of all ages

## Physical Activity Goal

- At least 30 minutes a day for children
- At least 15 minutes of moderate intensity physical activity for adults
- Exercise is one of the most potent anti-aging tools and stress busters available

Children and adults will see and feel results quickly. This should encourage them to increase their levels of activity.

## Stress

We all experience some levels of stress ourselves. Let's face it; there are often changes in our lives that cause various levels of stress. A loss of a loved one, relocation, divorce, work, overload, children or, just life itself.

How you deal with stress as an individual will determine its impact on you and your loved ones.

Create balance in your life by paying attention to your needs in a positive way. These should include your needs; physical, intellectual, emotional, family, spiritual and social; this will be a great place to start.

There is an incredible amount of stress and as many as 3 out of 4 people in the US today state, they are frazzled.

Beating stress is necessary if you are going to survive in today's world. Stress is a major factor in obesity, many diseases including heart disease and high blood pressure and Type 2 diabetes, headache, insomnia, depression, anxiety, dementia and the aging process. Reducing or eliminating stress is an important part of the Balance Walking Way. There are many ways to do this, let's go over some approaches that could work for you.

In many cases stress is self influenced, possibly by simply living or longing for the past or anticipating the future; and can turn into a mind game trying to figure everything out and anticipate everything that may or may not happen. In many cases it is only our thoughts that distract us from what's really important or from enjoying the moment.

## Some simple ways to attack STRESS h

One of the most effective ways is exercise, drinking green or black tea or eating a small piece of dark chocolate, laughter is a great way to reduce and eliminate stress.

Believe it or not, laughing is good for you! A great reason to enjoy a good laugh is that it actually instantaneously produces health benefits.

Some quiet time for yourself; as little as 5 minutes a day of quiet, where you think of nothing at all; this is form of meditation. You can actually meditate if you so choose. Try yoga, tai chi, listening to calming music, doing anything that takes the edge off and gives your mind a break from reality.

Stop focusing on the negative and think about the positive. Negative people have a way of pulling everyone down and the worst thing is, you cannot change them. Are you getting enough sleep? Do you have a strong social support network you can confide in? Sometimes just talking about it helps.

Everyone gets pulled in too many different directions – family, work, house, community to name a few. Most people are overwhelmed; we are way too busy chasing the dream that very few of us are enjoying the trip. By the way, the journey is what everything is about.

If you are a procrastinator stay focused, and start selecting each task that needs to be completed and accomplish them one at a time.

At work if you are overwhelmed, delegate. You can't do everything yourself even if you believe that you are the only one who can do it. On those tasks you need to get done, focus on the most important one first. Most people put off the most important task that needs to get done filling their time with less priority work, by prioritizing and staying focused, this will reduce the source of stress substantially.

DON'T BE A STRESS EATER; you will pack on pounds and for some reason stress poundage accumulates at your belly this is the most unhealthy place to pack it on.

There are many articles and studies now available on the direct relationship between stress and excessive weight gain as well, as loss. In addition, there are a number of studies relating stress to many illnesses. Although this makes sense, many of us are unaware of how to relieve this burden by minimizing stress to prevent such health problems.

The answer: Think positive instead of negative. How long do you think it took me to come up with that one? How simple could it be? Think about it; just look around you at the people you know. We all know at least one person that, for some reason, deals with one life crisis after another. But when you look closer they are constantly either thinking or talking negative. It seems their worst fears just continue to happen. Then there are the chosen ones. Everything they seem to do just works out, they are always positive and take the downside in stride, but seem to turn even negative events into positive ones. There is actually a bigger theory here and again, it is very simple. Be careful what you ask for because you might get it. But you can't just ask for it; you must believe it. I'm talking about a way of life. It may not show up tomorrow, but if you are positive enough, it will happen.

This all started with stress and how stress impacts a person's life. The Balance Walking Way also includes some suggestions on how to make stress reduction a regular part of your life.

Achieving wellness in ones life is not difficult; let's start with common sense and take ownership of your life. Our stressful lifestyles contribute significantly to the fix we are in today. Part of the fifteen minutes a day must be dedicated to stress reduction. Fortunately Balance Walking itself, especially if you do meditative walking, could have a big impact on your stress levels.

Some additional add-on techniques include taking some quiet time for yourself, it could be yoga, tai chi, meditation or, even more simply, just some quiet time. Just 5 minutes a day can have a very effective calming impact on your stress levels.

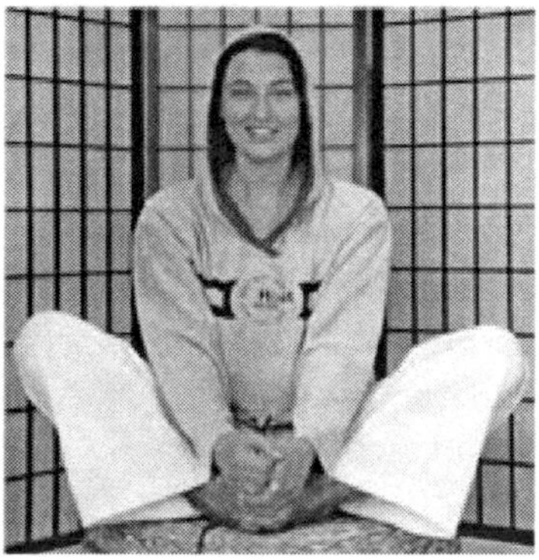

Here is a simple way to get started:

1. Find a peaceful place to sit and relax. Play soft meditative music or sounds of nature, the ocean, brook or even rain, whatever is what is relaxing to you.

2. Breathe slowly in and out. Try belly breathing like a baby – let your stomach rise and fall with each breath. First inhale deeply through your nose filling your lungs from the bottom up. Start with your belly, then mid lungs, then finally upper lungs. Hold for several seconds, then release. Exhale reversing the process. This may feel odd at first but you will easily get the rhythm.

3. Close your eyes and try not to think about anything but the moment. For me, thinking about floating in water is most effective, while some people like to float in air. What is important here is you are not thinking about anything. Sometimes a mantra will help or even a repetitive prayer. It simply puts your mind, in a suspense-like state.

4. When I finish a session, I like to rub my hands together to warm them up, then, place them over my eyes. It is a simple way to end the session while feeling very relaxing and energizing at the same time.

On stress busting, there are many ways you can approach this. Be optimistic and positive in the way you act and think; it works. Learn to accept life when a situation is out of your control, learn to let it go. Focus on the things you can change.

Part of your Balance Walking routine can be a reflective walk by yourself once or twice a week in a peaceful setting for you. It could simply be sitting for 5 to 10 minutes while allowing your mind to settle into a tranquil state. Some people listen to soothing sounds of nature, some people may repeat a prayer or a mantra; these approaches all have the same effect on the mind. If you want to really open your mind, you may consider going traditional with one of the many forms of meditation. Tai chi is considered a moving meditation with low impact, non-combative movements to build strength and create structural balance in the body. The list is endless; the point is to take a few minutes everyday. Let's say 5 minutes of quiet time. You can test the calming effects of meditation very simply. Start in a comfortable position, in a quiet or serene place that is dimly lit or shaded. At this time you may not want to lie down because sleeping is not meditation. The process starts with relaxed breathing as described earlier, as you start to relax, gently close your eyes and continue the breathing and relaxing for 5 to 10 minutes. You may use a mantra or sound to keep you focused in the moment. When thoughts wander in let them move through, do not dwell on them. Sometimes picturing yourself floating through the air or water will help bring you back. If you use a mantra continue to repeat it slowly in your mind.

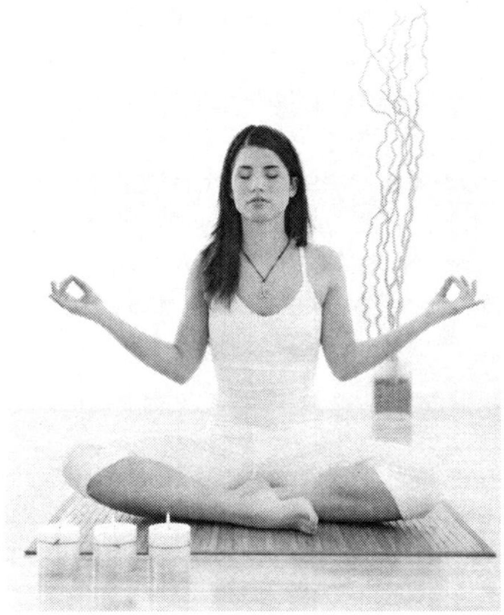

As you end your meditation or quiet time, wind down slowly, rub your hands together and place the palms over your eyes before opening them. Feel the warmth of your palms, soothing and relaxing, then, wipe your face with your hands while feeling the warmth and glow of your own body.

It sounds crazy but it works as a healing process that will substantially reduce stress and give you a new energy and life.

When I was in college, I was working 50 hours a weeks and going to school fulltime on a scholarship that I had to maintain a 3.2 average to keep. I was married and had a baby daughter so I did not have any choice but to support my family while trying to achieve my goals and dreams.

During my last semester I realized I needed to get an A in all 5 courses to graduate Magna Cum Laude, I stressed myself to the limit. My doctor told me I was developing ulcers and could not continue to push my body like I had been and that I really needed more than 4-5 hours sleep if I wanted to live to enjoy my children.

The following week I was introduced to transcendental meditation (T.M.) on the campus at the University of New Haven. I practiced meditation everyday for 15 minutes and within a matter of weeks I was able to de-stress myself and yes, I aced my 5 courses and accomplished my dream. That is, until the next dream came along.

That was back when I was a very young man. Today I would handle that situation differently but that is some of the wisdom that comes with age. The point is, meditation and quiet time work and are great ways for you to refocus your energy and stomp out stress.

Today I still push myself to the limit but when I need to I will shut my office door and find a quiet place in my mind that washes away my stress. Time to say 'omm' or use whatever sound is right for you. This works great and is an important part of the Balance Walking program.

Can't handle the meditation side? Don't like the quiet walks? Then turn to other forms of mediation in movement, tai chi or yoga, to increase your flexibility and help to relax your mind.

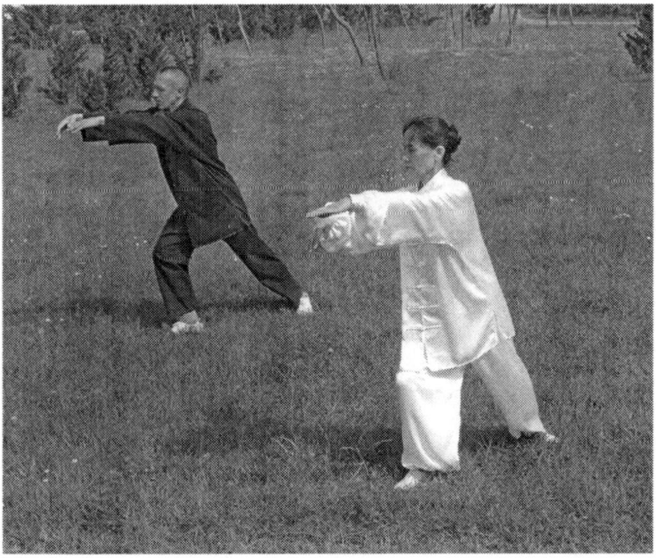

With yoga and tai chi, there is no strain; you work to the level that is right for your body. People well into their 80's are performing tai chi daily, as it forms a beautiful, slow dance based on the martial arts. These forms of mind and body control and relaxation have been around for centuries. Look to the wisdom of the Far East. If they did not work, people would not still be doing them.

**Benefits are:**

### 1. Healthy Body

- Develop physical power
- Improve strength and flexibility
- Manage weight
- Relieve pain
- Sleep better
- Stimulate the immune system
- Lowers blood pressure and cholesterol levels
- Slows the heart rate
- Reverses the effects of aging

### 2. Happy Mind

- Find emotional serenity
- Release stress
- Become centered and balanced
- Reverse depression and anxiety
- Improve focus and concentration

### 3. Peaceful Spirit

- Awaken spiritual energy
- Increase self-awareness and self-acceptance
- Foster inner joy and happiness
- Enhance personal relationships
- Discover inner peace

## Muscle Mass & Strength

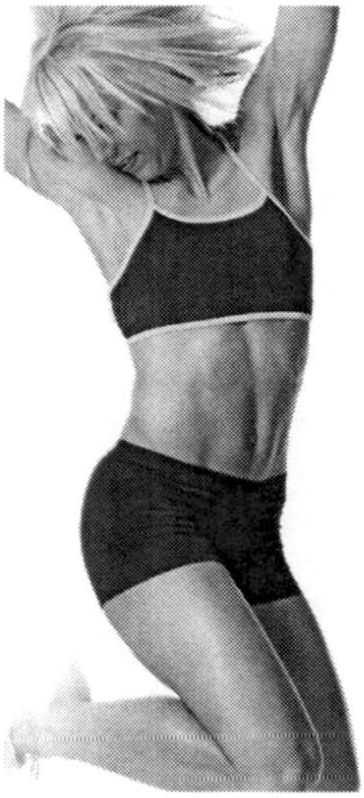

The fountain of youth and the key to feeling and looking young is muscle mass and tone. Everyone, regardless of age, should focus on developing muscular strength, endurance, cardiovascular fitness and flexibility. The absolute wonderful part of the body is its ability to regain muscle mass, shape and toning at any age. It is important to incorporate our recommended strength training into your Balance Walking Way program. Strength training is done 2 to 3 times per week.

We recommend a modified version of the Kettlebell routine. Jeff Hopeck, United States Secret Service veteran, has partnered with Balance Walking author, Raymond Margiano, to provide a Kettlebell routine designed to focus on fast weight loss, strength training and heart health. This routine will only take 15 minutes and will produce results with only 2 to 3 sessions per week.

For the first time Jeff Hopeck has created a training routine that fits today's busy adult who is looking for a quick, healthy, weight loss solution. Whether the goal is to lose a lot of weight or shed those last few pounds, Hopeck's unique Kettlebell training method is not only effective, but time saving and very safe to perform. The cardio and muscle strengthening workout is combined into one routine that can be done in half the time compared to walking on a treadmill resulting in faster weight loss.

Joseph Doughty, D.C. of ProSport Wellness & Chiropractic, tried them out himself. Not only did he save time and achieve results, Doughty noted that the program is safe, effective and easy making even the beginner feel comfortable. Doughty commented "My endurance has doubled and my strength increased 40% in just two and a half months. I could never be this cut and lean in the past without very closely watching my diet." The exercises are quick, simple and effective.

## 1. Swing:

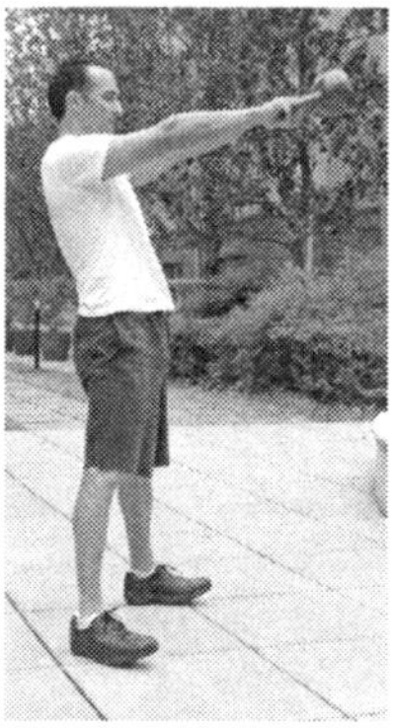

Begin in a relaxed athletic stance, holding the jeffHopeck Bellä between your legs; drive your hips forward to begin momentum, and swing the bell to forehead height. Keep your weight on your heels and your abs contracted. Continue this in a repeated motion just like a pendulum.

## 2. Squat/Bell Row:

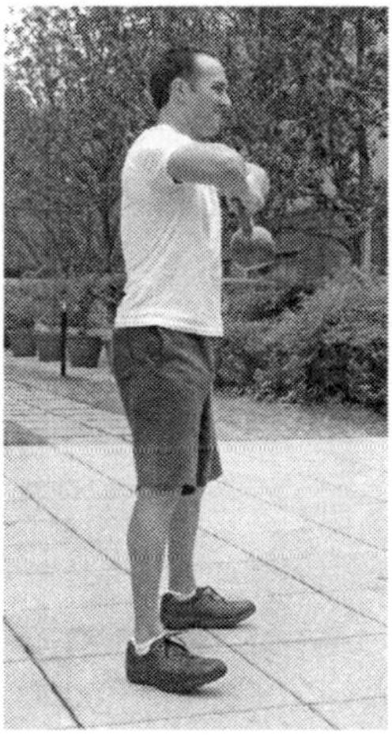

Begin in a low squat stance, holding the jeffHopeck Bellä with two hands, bell low to the ground (Keep your back slightly bent, but STRAIGHT and SUPPORTED. Avoid hunching over so that your back looks like the letter "C"). This position loads the hamstrings, quads, and glutes for the exercise. Drive up on your heels, perform an upright row pulling the bell upwards, keeping it close to your body.

## 3. Compound Curl:

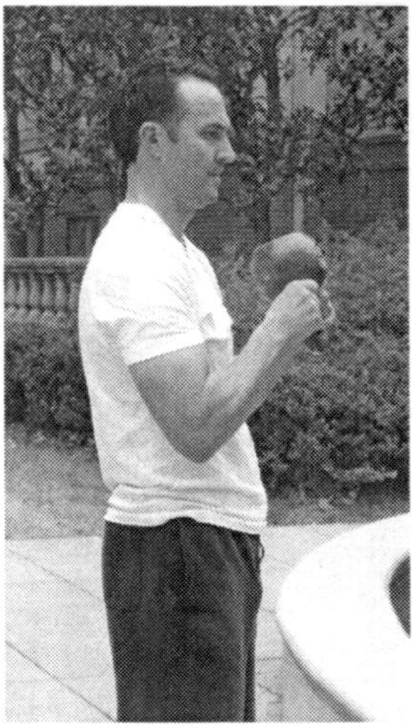

Begin by holding the jeffHopeck Bellä by the handles, resting your arms over the upper thighs. Perform the curl, keeping you elbows close to your sides, and abs contracted (supporting your lower back). Lower the jeffHopeck Bellä to the starting position using a steady, controlled motion.

Balance Walking includes all the basics needed to change your life with only the demand of 15 minutes everyday. The program goals are clear – safe, core muscle workouts that increase strength, endurance and cardiovascular performance while having fun. The result is healthy weight loss and improved muscle tone. Once again, the combination of Kettlebell training and Balance Walking delivers results faster than anything else.

## Balance Walking

The Balance Walking coaches and website will provide detailed information on the Kettlebell/Balance Walking system with a direct links to Jeff Hopeck's website and a specialized Kettlebell training program designed to compliment the Balance Walking system.

Your Chung Shi shoes will increase your Kettlebell workout results according to Jeff Hopeck based on his own experience with this specialty shoe.

## Set Your Goals

Challenge yourself – don't forget to vary your routine, otherwise it will become just that - a boring routine leading to burn out and muscle memory retention which, in turn, will reduce the results of your program. Setting short and long-term, realistic and challenging goals will work, and changing up your routine will increase you potential success.

The retention of muscle mass and the reversing of traditional loss of muscle mass: The average male loses 30% of their muscle mass from age 20 to 70. It not only effects the way we feel but it adds to the slow down of the body and metabolism. Muscle mass burns more calories and keeps the fire burning. This is an area you cannot ignore, take your clothes off and look into the mirror. Take a good look, noticing where you are sagging or starting to sag. Toning and shaping will give new life to how you look and feel. Combine this firming and shaping with improved body alignment; a by product of the Chung Shi shoes and Balance Walking program. Your friends and family will notice the difference, you will look and feel years younger and all for a small investment of only 15 minutes per day.

Optional alternatives include power yoga; check out yoga-doc.com the website of Dr. Craig Aaron. I have attended his classes and Dr. Aaron's version of power yoga will improve your flexibility and reshape your body. With just a couple of postures he will put your body in melt down mode.

If you had to choose one yoga exercise then I would strongly recommend the Salutation to the SUN (Soorya Namaskar). The Sun is considered to be the deity for health and longevity. The Sun experience will bring back lost flexibility and take you through 12 positions. You can do this in normal yoga form or be more aggressive with power yoga; the choice is yours. There are many sources and instructors available for basic yoga techniques if you are interested in this area.

Other options include simple exercises, lightweight routines, resistance training, Pilates, etc. - anything that will work your muscles enough to force your body to do some rebuilding. The glorious part here is that you can mix this up; shock your muscles by hitting them from every angle. Remember we are elongating muscles as well as improving flexibility. We are creating a body for fluid movement and longevity. Visit our website for suggestions and different exercises to help change up your program and keep it interesting.

Carrying extra weight increases your risk not only for heart disease, but for physical injuries to your feet, legs and back as well. As one reaches middle age the average person will lose about one pound a year of muscle mass, usually replacing it with fat cells. Strength training will reduce your waistline and critical belly fat. The rate at which your body burns calories slows down as you age; this is another reason why eating smaller meals more often and reducing calorie intake as we age is critical for winning the battle of the bulge.

Regular exercise also serves as a detoxification method. The lymphatic system is being flushed and cells are being flooded with health giving oxygen. You can also detox by including a teaspoon of apple cider vinegar everyday in a glass of water, an alternative would be lemon juice in a glass of water.

Use a sauna as a dry-heat sweat bath. Sweating helps rid the body of toxins and excess water, regulates body temperature and invigorates the body's largest organ, the skin. One thing is clear, in order to maintain balance you need to follow the complete program; one healthy behavior without the others will not work, you need to maintain all four of the Balance Walking program segments to change your lifestyle and maintain the desired long-term results.

## Support for the Active Foot

In athletics, there is a greater importance placed on balance, support, performance and endurance of your feet. You can improve your game by combining the right shoe insert, socks and properly fitted shoes for every sport, from golfing to skiing to running.

What you wear on your feet is the most important part of proper foot care. Many problems, such as aches in your feet, ankles, knees, lower back and even your shoulders, stem from improper treatment of your feet. These pains are often caused simply by the style and fit of your shoes. A supportive shoe, combined with the proper insert, will put your foot into its natural position for walking, standing and training.

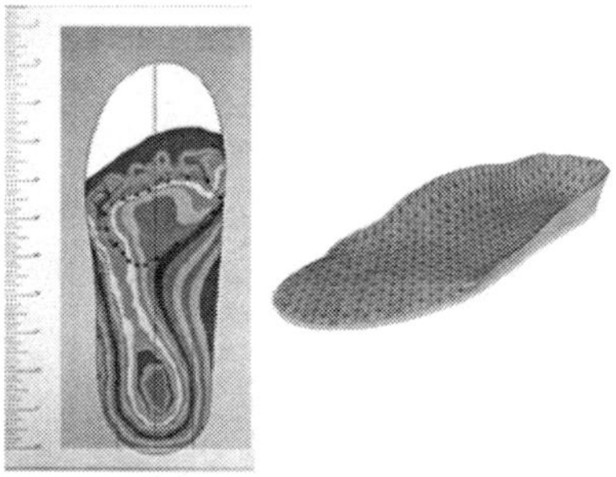

Custom Arch Supports
Using Todays Technology

By putting your foot in balance, the alignment of other joints will be improved. Taking care of your feet is taking care of the whole you.

However, there are athletic problems you should be aware of and look out for. They include:

## Achilles Tendonitis

Symptoms: Pain and tightness felt in the lower calf muscles, which may be more prevalent in the morning.

Causes: Constant hill running, shoes with soft heel counters, switching from dress shoes to running shoes.

Solutions: Ice massage, calf stretches, proper rest, softer running surface, update your shoes often, paying attention to the heel.

## Bunions

Symptoms: Aches are felt around the big toe and a noticeable lump at the first metatarsal joint. Usually, the big toe angles toward the other toes in an abnormal fashion.

Causes: Heredity, wearing shoes that are too tight across the ball of the foot.

Solutions: Wear shoes with a wider toe area. If area is red and holds a temperature, consult your physician.

## Hip Pain/Bursitis

Symptoms: Pain on the outer hip area and near the buttocks muscles. The hip joint has a large bursa sac (a sac that contains fluid used to lubricate and protect the joint), which can become inflamed.

Causes: Structural weaknesses, overuse and trauma (such as child birth, a fall, etc.)

Solutions: Change your activities to adjust, use ice, massage and stretching. If pain is felt in buttocks or legs, consult your physician.

## Illiotibial Band Syndrome (ITB)

Symptoms: A type of sharp, burning knee or upper leg pain that afflicts many runners.

Causes: When the band thickens and rubs over the femur bone (thigh bone), the area can become inflamed, or the band itself may become irritated. Either occurrence can cause a common knee injury's characteristic of a sharp burning pain.

Solutions: Combine simple exercises, deep massage and specific ITB stretching.

## Morton's Neuroma

Symptoms: Pain, burning, tingling or numbness that occurs between the third and fourth toes and in the ball of your foot; may be caused by a growth around the nerves.

Causes: Collapse of the arch, heredity, obesity and wearing shoes that are too tight.

Solutions: An arch support with a metatarsal pad to support the foot, customized as needed.

## Plantar Fasciitis

Symptoms: Pain felt along the bottom of the foot from the heel to the arch. Often felt more in the morning and at the end of the day.

Causes: Standing for long periods at a time, obesity, having one leg longer than the other, wearing unsupportive shoes, calf and Achilles tightness.

Solutions: Arch supports, night splints and a stretching program combined with early diagnosis to provide relief.

### Runner's Knee

Symptoms: Pain felt often below the kneecap, which increases while walking up stairs or at an incline or sitting for long periods of time. Frequently found in adolescent runners.

Causes: Flat feet, weak thigh muscles, and insufficient rest between exercising.

Solutions: Beyond simply making sure that you're getting enough rest so that your muscles can heal after exercising, arch supports along with an ice massage can really make a difference.

### Shin Splints

Symptoms: Sharp pain felt around the shinbone. It is very common in people who exercise too much, too soon (beginners especially), and too fast. Untreated shin splints can become painful stress fractures.

Causes: Calf and Achilles tightness due to lack of appropriate stretching before and after exercising. Also, unsupportive or worn out shoes.

Solutions: Ice massage, supportive shoes, and a softer running surface can help relieve shin splints.

## What To Do If Your Feet Are Hurting

Consult your nearest Foot Solutions store or sports medicine professional about any pain you are experiencing before it creates more problems.

Replace your shoes often (usually between 200 - 450 miles). Take your worn shoes to a Foot Solutions consultant for a full analysis of your potential problems.

Ice massage, using an item such as a cold plastic soda bottle, does wonders for a painful arch.

An ice pack for pain in hips, back and knees, as well as shin splints and Achilles' tendon problems also works well.

## Did you know?

The average person walks the equivalent of 3.5 times around the world during his/her lifetime.

Ninety Percent of all people wear improperly fitted shoes. Ouch!

The human foot contains twenty-six bones, thirty-three joints and over one hundred tendons, muscles and ligaments. That's an awful lot of places for pain to occur.

Most foot problems are caused or aggravated by poorly fitted shoes.

## Some basic tips on fitting

It is best to be fitted by a trained Pedorthist especially if you have any fitting issues. Most people are in improperly fitted shoes and most people don't really know what a properly fitted shoe should feel like. Hint – if it does not feel right in the shoe store it is not going to get better, in fact in most cases it will get worse.

If your feet are hurting you will not be balance walking or enjoying many activities at all.

**Some tips on how to fit your feet properly:**

Forget about what shoe size and width you think you are.

Whenever trying on shoes always get both feet measured.

Remember shoe sizes vary from manufacturer and style – you must try them on.

We all have difficult shaped feet – choose a shoe that is a match for your foot shape.

Shoes should be as wide as your feet and at least 3/7 to 1/2 inch longer.

The widest part of your foot is called 'the ball' and should fit in the widest part of the shoe and match the flex point for your feet.

Heels must fit comfortably in the shoe, not too tight or loose.

Your feet change in size and shape depending on activity level and time of day, so take this into consideration when getting fitted.

Walk in the shoe at least around the store or at home on the carpet to insure a proper fit.

If you wear inserts or orthotics they will also impact the way a shoe fits. Make sure the new shoe is designed to accommodate the insert or orthotic.

Poorly fitted shoes can cause bunions, corns, calluses, hammertoes and other foot problems. Let's start by taking care of your feet with properly fitted shoes. You only have one pair and they must last you a life time.

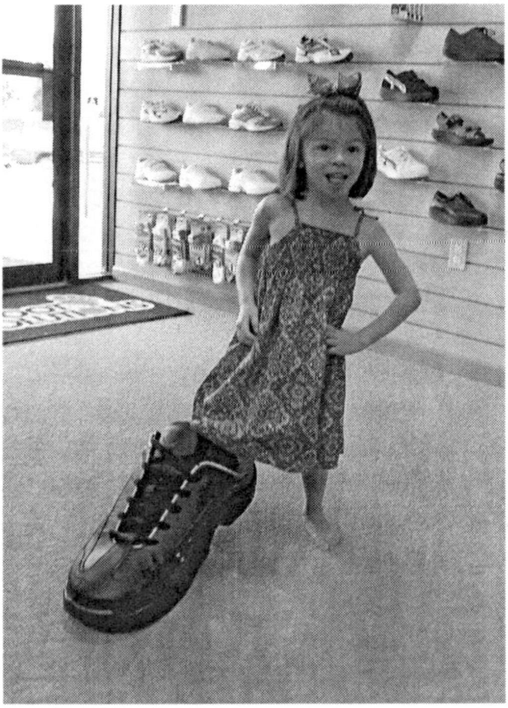

## Socks

We discussed properly fitted shoes and how important it is to have the right size and shaped shoe.

For Balance walking my sock of choice is Padds by Thorlo, this sock is designed to cushion the fatty pad areas on the bottom of your feet that get worn out and displaced as we age and exercise. Socks are a major part of an integrated solution for your individual feet along with shoes and properly designed arch supports. Some people are concerned about thickness of socks or pads making their feet too hot. Usually the feeling of hot or cold feet is caused by improper fitting shoes and/or socks. This is why I mention the integrated product system solution. The proper thickness of the sock and properly fitted shoes allows a more complete range of motion of the feet, at the same time protecting against friction and chafing from the inside of the shoe.

This approach helps to stimulate circulation in the feet while the sock helps provide insulation and air flow, which helps moderate temperature and keeps the feet from getting too hot or too cold. Make socks part of your complete exercise package.

## Dressing for Balance Walking

Shoes and socks are special and have been covered in more detail in chapter 20.

Nordic pole walking can be done in all kinds of weather but you must dress accordingly.

- Dress in layers
- Wear clothes that breathe
- Loose fitting

You will want to dress so you will be comfortable and not get chilled. Especially when first starting to warm up or even walking or driving to your trail area.

Important: Once you start walking you will get warm. Depending on weather and conditions as you warm up if dressed in layers you can take a layer off. Remember as you slow down and before you cool off make sure you put your extra layer back on, this makes common sense and will prevent chill.

Layering is important especially in colder weather. When cross country skiing in the winter in upstate New York I learned very quickly that layering is critical.

In the dead of winter when you are really sweating, when you stop skiing if you don't have a layer to put on you will chill down very rapidly. Cross country skiing can be extreme if you want it to be, watch the Olympics, you can see the cross country skiers and teams pushing themselves to the limit and total exhaustion. This is a huge sport in Europe and the rivalries are very high between countries.

Nordic pole walking is not nearly as extreme but for those of you that do push yourselves dressing properly and taking care not to get chilled is important. Remember Nordic pole walking is for fun and for you to enjoy yourself, to become one with nature and yourself or to enjoy the companionship of a partner or group.

**Pedometer** - here you can get a basic pedometer to a sophisticated unit that will down load into your computer. You need to be interested in time and distance. Most simple pedometers will give you number of steps, distance walked and in some cases calories burned. For Balance walking you are interested in amount of time and distance covered.

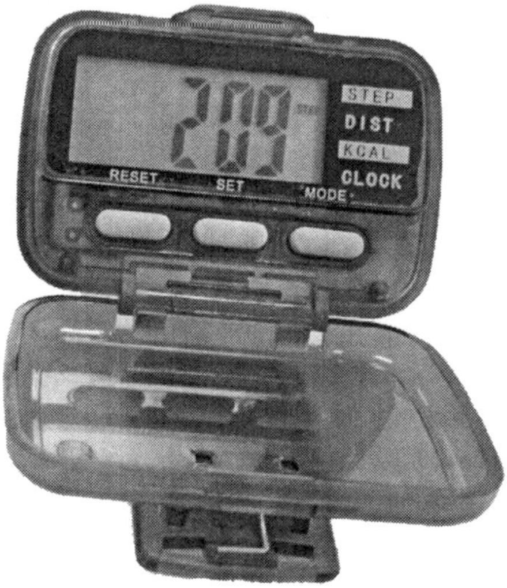


To make something effective and long lasting like a life style change you must make it part of your body habit. Do this for 6 to 8 weeks every day and you will start the habit forming process.

To start with you want to make a commitment of 15 minutes every day for this program. FIFTEEN MINUTES A DAY!

Carve 15 minutes out that is best for you - morning, lunch, evening. My suggestion is to make if part of your routine earlier in the day. For most people the end of the day seems to take on a life of it's own with new priorities pulling you away from your schedule.

The key here is the time of the day that you can consistently devote 15 minutes everyday, this actually is very easy to accomplish, no matter how hectic your schedule is.

Start by planning your weekly/monthly routine. You must start with 15 minutes Balance walking every day for at least 4 to 6 weeks. You can then add some of the other components to your routine. You can mix up the components to very your routine but you must Balance walk at least 4 times per week.

As you establish the routine that is best for you, two 15 minute sessions should be dedicated to retaining or rebuilding muscle mass and definition. Here I strongly recommend the 15 minute Kettlebell routine designed for the Balance walking program. Alternates could be yoga or any effective muscle resistance program you enjoy.

If time is critical to your schedule and you can only dedicate 15 minutes a day then save at least one session for mind relaxation and stress busting meditation. This would be better achieved if you took just 5 minutes a day, say mid-afternoon or whatever is best for your quiet time.

Since eating is the 4th cornerstone of Balance walking try simplifying, eating smaller meals and snacks more often through the day. Enjoy what you eat it is one of the simple pleasures of life, but don't abuse it.

## Time and Distance

At the beginning forget about distance. Depending on your physical shape and level of activity walk to a pace that is comfortable for you. Don't forget a minimum of 15 minutes per day, do this for several weeks then introduce distance either using a pedometer or walking measured areas – the magic number is one mile.

If you are not physically fit you will probably take 30 minutes to walk a mile. Let's start by working that time down to 15 minute miles. For females in great shape and pushing the envelope you can get down to 12 minutes per mile, for men 10 minute miles. Remember this is not about speed or killing yourself, walk to a pace right for you. Your body will send you signals, this is all about consistency and making it part of your daily personal routine. Joining walking clubs or classes will help participate in events. Walk with your family, at work at lunchtime, at the mall before mall hours, if you are travelling, take your poles and use them.

## Personal Log

At the beginning until your specific Balance walking program has become a way of life for you, I recommend keeping a personal journal.

Log your activities in daily

1. Time and distance walked on each day – remember your personal goal of a minimum of 15 minutes.

2. Meditation time.

3. Resistance time.

4. Flexibility.

5. Food – list food, water, number of meals.

This process is to help you identify where to make adjustments, this is not a diet, it is slowly changing what you do to enjoy eating but also putting it in balance.

This simple daily log will help you track what you are accomplishing and will also help build consistency and positive habits that will make the Balance Walking Way a permanent part of your life.

## A simple example – my daily log

7:30 - Breakfast – 1 egg with 2 egg whites scrambled, whole grain toast, glass of grapefruit juice (1/2 juice, ½ water)

8:30 – 15 minute Nordic pole walk – I mile

9:00 - Glass of water

10:30 – Snack – yogurt drink

12:30 – Lunch – salad with grilled chicken, glass of water with teaspoon of apple cider vinegar

3:00 – Snack – apple/string cheese, glass of water

4:00 – 5 minute meditation

5:00 – Glass of water

6:30 Dinner – grilled salmon, sautéed garlic spinach, cup of cantaloupe, glass of water

9:00 – Cup of herbal tea

Note: This is just a simple way to track what you are doing. I did not mention portion size in my journal but if this is an issue for you, make sure you include portion sizes.

Visit www.balancewalking.com for recommendations on different routines, references for different meals and portion controls you can live with. Blogs, coaches, free introductory classes, events and participation in Presidents Challenge program.

# References

1. Nordic Pole Walking burns up to 46% more calories that exercise walking without poles or moderate jogging. (Cooper Institute, 2004, Dallas and other). Extremely great weight loss program in combination with conscious nutrition.

2. Increases heart and cardiovascular training to 22% more effect (Foley 1994, Jordan 2001, Morss t al., 2001 and other).

3. Incorporates 90% of all body muscles in one exercise and increases endurance of arm muscles (triceps) and neck and shoulder muscles (Latissmus) to 38% (Karawan et al., 1992 and other).

4. Eliminates back, shoulder and neck pain (Attila et al., 1999 and other).

5. Less impact on hip, knee and foot joints about 26% (Wilson et al., 2001 and other).

6. Increase production of "positive" hormones. Decreases "negative" hormones (R.M. Klatz et. Al., 1999; Dharma Singh Khalsa 1997).

7. Supports stress management and mental disorders (Stoughton 1992, Momment-Jauch, 2003).

8. Human Performance Laboratory, University of Calgary, Bio-Mechanics of walking in the Chung Shi health shoe, October, 2006.

9. National Consumer Research 2005, Finland. Research article on Nordic pole walking and health benefits.

10. New German fitness trend makes strides 2005.

11. Research on results on responses to pole walking training published in 1992 by Stoughton, Sarken and Kareven from the University of Oregon.

12. Effect of Chung Shi walking shows on posture, foot shape, balance, flexibility, menstruation, pain, body composition, and gait, EWHA Women's University, Gait Biomechanics Laboratory, Yi Kyung OK, November, 2006.

## About the Author

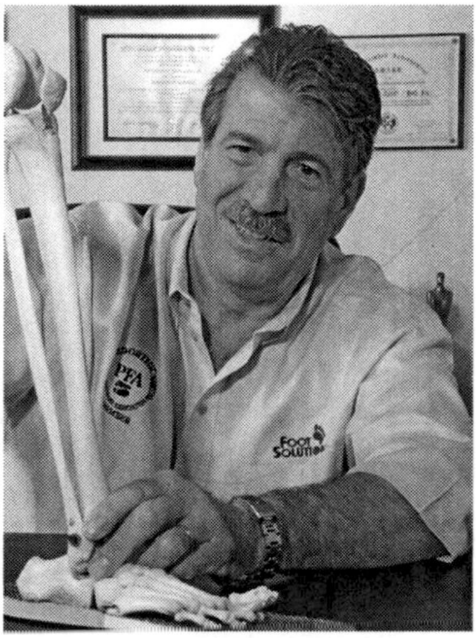

Ray Margiano PhD, Pedorthist, Entrepreneur and Founder and CEO of Foot Solutions, Inc, the largest retail pedorthic group in the world; focusing on Health & Wellness and proper support for the feet.

As an international business person and entrepreneur with huge demands on my time, at the end of the day there was just nothing left for me. Balance walking combines the best of what I could come up with based on my world wide exposure and interest in a healthy living style, time being the most critical element in this equation. Balance walking only requires an investment of 15 minutes a day; the catch is a life time commitment. The four elements include the walking segment, stress reduction, healthy eating and building/retaining muscle mass. This is a simple program for everyone interested in gaining enormous benefits that will change the way you look, feel and live. This low impact approach can save millions of dollars in medical costs and help you live a fuller happier life.

Sound too good to be true? Balance walking is the combination of proven methods that have stood the test of time. Now it is up to you to turn back the clock.

Part of the funds raised from the sale of this book will be used for continuing studies and research on the impact of Balance walking on diabetic patients, heart problems and obesity.

LaVergne, TN USA
09 October 2009

160395LV00001B/2/P

9 780615 190884